Cognitive exercises

99

Activities
& Games

for Seniors with
Dementia & Alzheimer

Very easy & relaxing

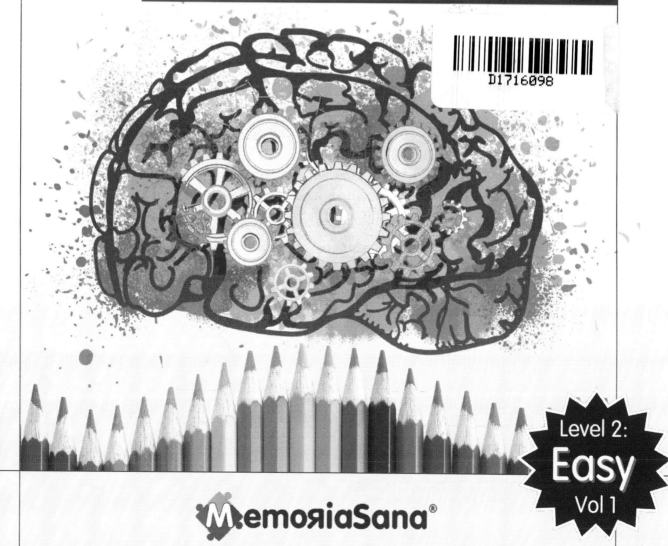

Level 2:
Easy
Vol 1

MemoriaSana®

99 Cognitive Exercises, Activities & Games for Seniors with Dementia & Alzheimer. Memory Activity Book Large Print. Very Easy & Relaxing

Produced by: Memoriasana

www.memoriasana.com

Design and edited by: Memoriasana

This workbook belongs to ...

....

Who lives in this address ...

....

....

....

It was started on ...

....

It was finished on ...

....

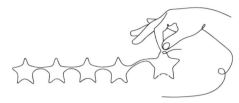

YOUR FEEDBACK MEANS SO MUCH TO US...

We want to sincerely thank you for trusting us by choosing this book. Your support and confidence are the driving force that inspires us to continue developing high-quality products that truly improve people's lives. We hope you enjoy each activity and find moments of joy and connection along the way.

We truly wish you had a great time with this experience! It would mean a lot to us if you could take a moment to leave a review. Not only will it help us as independent authors, but it will also help others find and enjoy these activities too.

https://amzn.to/479LSeC

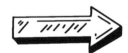

How would you rate it?

☆☆☆☆☆

Share a video or photo

Title your review

What's most important to know?

Write your review

What did you like or dislike? What did you use this product for?

Submit

Together, we'll make cognitive wellness a reality!

WE PROMOTE COGNITIVE HEALTH

Our mission is to give you the tools that **support active and healthy aging**. We understand that keeping your mind engaged is essential for a fulfilling life, so we've created these fun mental activities just for you. Our goal is to offer exercises that not only **boost your cognitive skills** but also **bring you joy and relaxation**. We encourage you to check out our other difficulty levels tailored to suit different needs and help keep your mind sharp.

As a little thank you, we have a **special gift for you**: two books crafted to **enhance your cognitive well-being** and keep your **mind in shape**. Download them and keep learning while enjoying more activities made for your well-being.

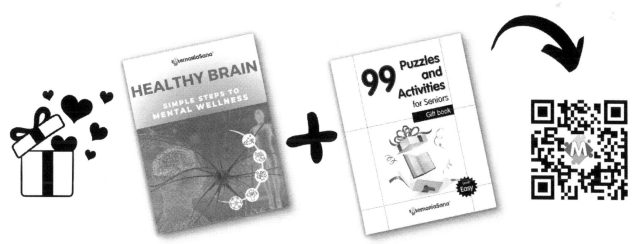

https://bit.ly/Easy-Gift

You can also drop us a message at **comercial@memoriasana.com**, and we'll send it to you. Just mention **Easy Level**!

Thanks a bunch for your support!

Find us as MEMORIASANA, where you'll discover a variety of books and cognitive stimulation activities

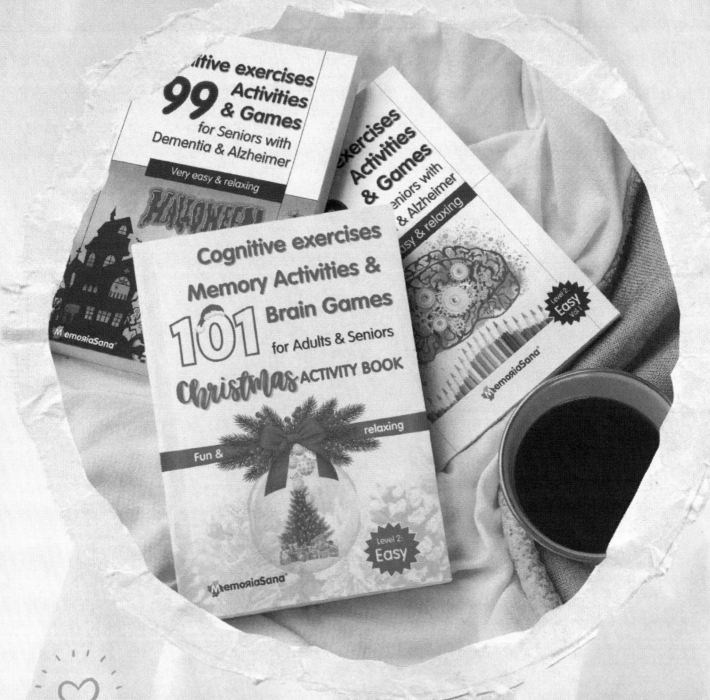

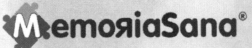

7 TIPS

in case you wish to accompany the realization in the book's activities

MAKE A CHEERFUL ENVIRONMENT:

Allocate a specific peaceful, cozy, and illuminated area for conducting activities.

SHARE THE EXPERIENCE:

Remember that each person progresses at their own pace; celebrate the small achievements.

BE PATIENT & POSITIVE:

Attitude is important. Stay patient and offer constant encouragement.

PROGRESS AT YOUR OWN PACE:

Remember that each person progresses at their own pace; celebrate the small achievements.

FIND YOUR FLOW:

It is advisable to do the activities in the book at the time of day when your beloved feels most lucid and active.

INVOLVES THE SENSES:

Accompany the sessions with relaxing music or aromas that can positively stimulate memory and concentration.

CELEBRATE ACHIEVEMENTS:

No matter how small, recognizing each step forward motivates and uplifts your spirit.

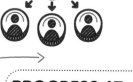

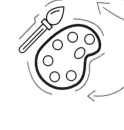

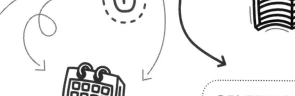

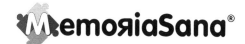

MemoriaSana®

FOR YOU TO KEEP IN MIND....

LEVEL OF DIFFICULTY: EASY ...

The activities of this book are intended for healthy elderly people of very advanced age or with cognitive impairment caused by dementia, such as moderate Alzheimer's disease.

THE ACTIVITIES ARE NOT LISTED IN ORDER...

You can do the exercises as you prefer, the book does not have a set order.

WORK ON YOUR OWN TIME...

Take your time, there is no rush to finish. What is expected is that you enjoy and relax while keeping your brain active.

ENGAGE DIFFERENT BRAIN AREAS ...

You can preserve and/or enhance a variety of cognitive abilities with the variety of activities, including reasoning, attention, memory, language, perception, problem solving, fine motor skills, mathematical logic, and attention among others.

AS WELL AS ....

HOW IT WORKS ...

Activities should challenge the brain and not be repetitive in order to increase your cognitive reserve and the connection between neurons.

CONSTANCY WINS...

30 to 60 minutes a day is enough to maintain your cognitive reserve. However, the more mental activity you have, the better your cognitive health will be.

OTHER NECESSARY HABITS ...

Practicing other habits, such as socializing with family and friends, engaging in physical activity, maintaining a healthy diet, getting enough sleep, etc.; are important for maintaining a good quality of life.

THE SOLUTIONS ARE AT THE END...

If you feel stuck, you can go to the end of the book, where you will find the solutions to the different exercises.

Select the shortest path so that Victoria can eat her snack:

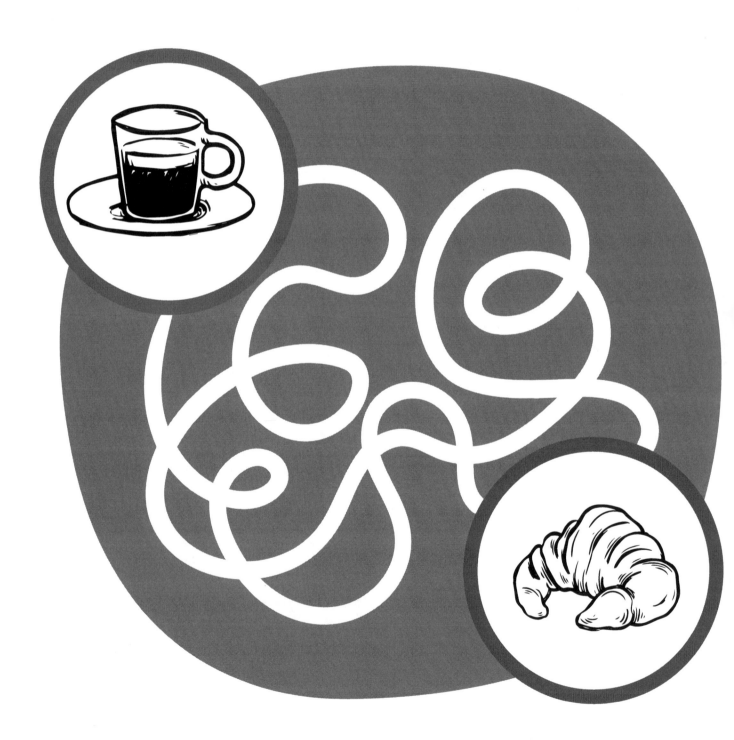

Date: ..../................/..............   Duration: ....

Start time: ....   End time: ....

Mark with an **X** the respective box according to the following instructions:

- To the left of this figure
- Below this figure
- Above this figure
- To the right of this figure

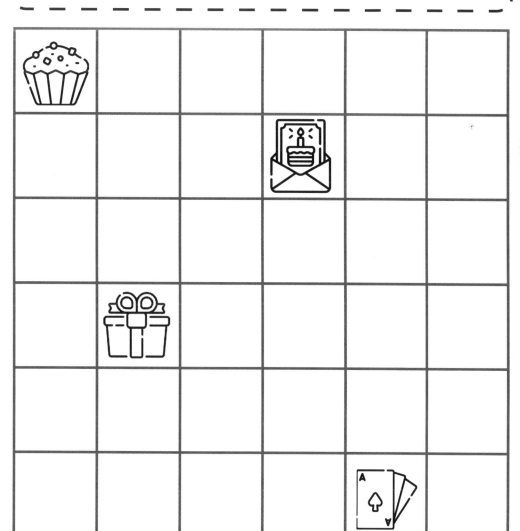

Date: ..../..................../..............   Duration: ....

Start time: ....   End time: ....

In each box, write the name of 10 objects according to the instructions:

Fruits

....

....

....

....

....

....

....

....

....

....

Vegetables

....

....

....

....

....

....

....

....

....

....

Date: ..../ ..../	Duration: ....
Start time:	End time: ....

Mark with an **X** the object that does NOT belong to the group:

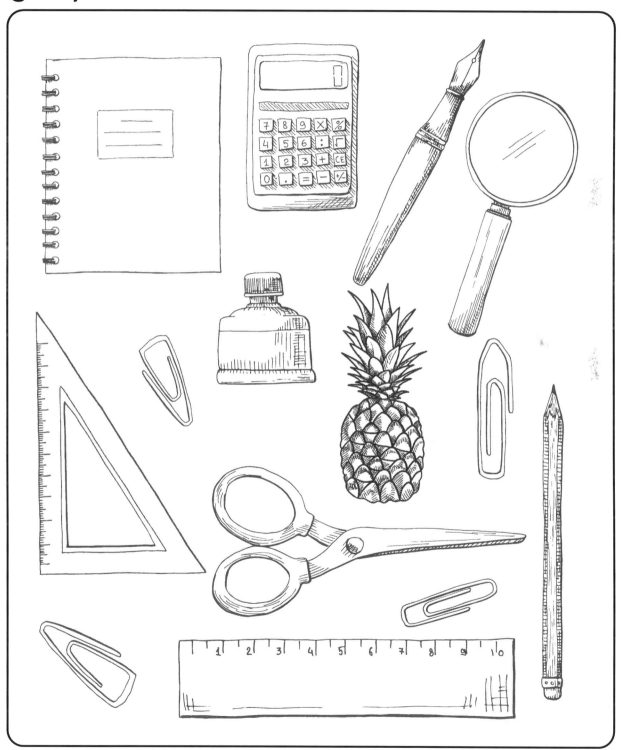

Date: ..../.............../............   Duration: ....

Start time: ....   End time: ....

Write the names of the objects in the box on the dotted line:

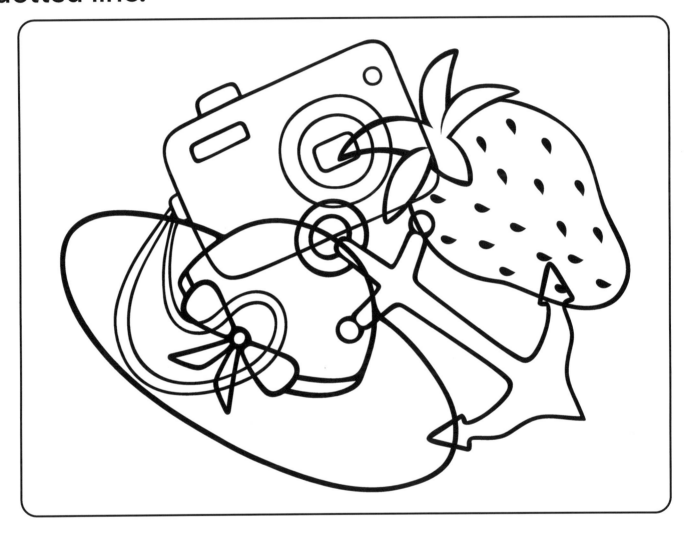

....

....

....

....

Date: ..../.............../..............

Duration: ....

Start time: ....

End time: ....

Write the numbers by twos until you reach 84:

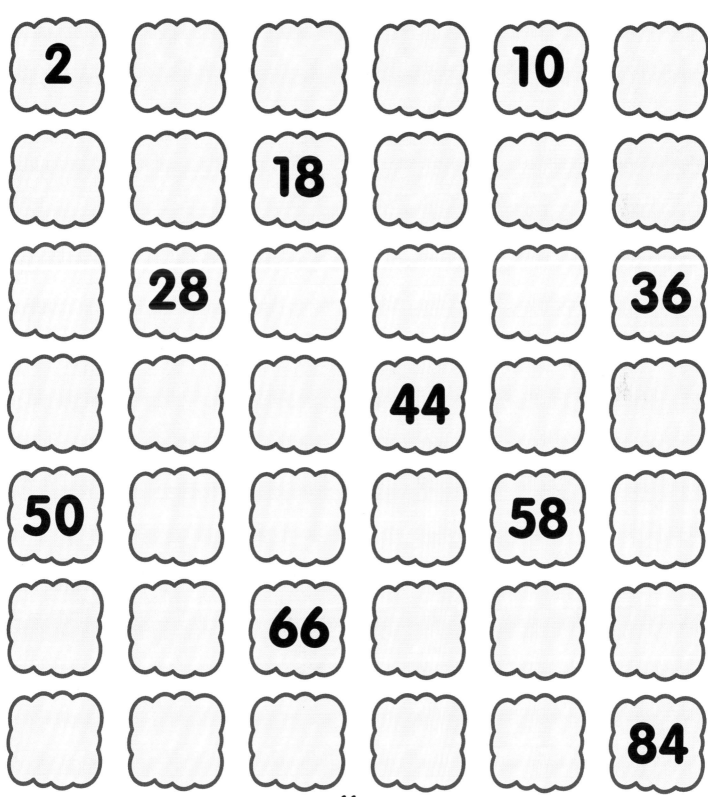

2   ___   ___   ___   10   ___

___   ___   18   ___   ___   ___

___   28   ___   ___   ___   36

___   ___   ___   44   ___   ___

50   ___   ___   ___   58   ___

___   ___   66   ___   ___   ___

___   ___   ___   ___   ___   84

Date: ..../.............../.............   Duration: ....

Start time: ....   End time: ....

Mark the incorrect box with an X:

6 four	8 eight	7 seven
4 four	9 three	1 one
3 six	2 two	0 nine

Date: ..../.............../.............   Duration: ....

Start time: ....   End time: ....

Reproduce the drawing in the box below:

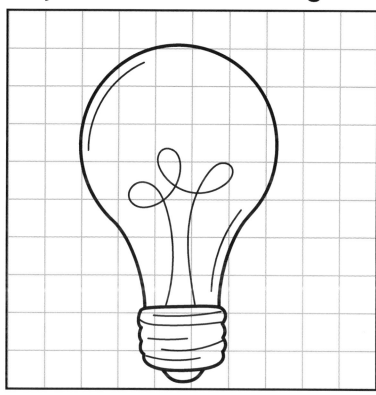

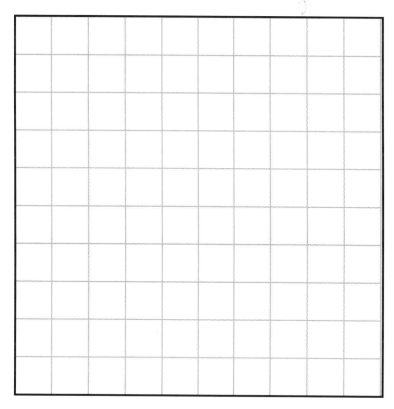

Date: ..../.............../.............

Duration: ....

Start time: ....

End time: ....

Answer the questions:

TO REMEMBER IS TO LIVE AGAIN...

¿Where were you born?

....

¿In what year were you born?

....

¿What were your parents' names?

....

....

¿How many siblings did you have?

....

¿What were the names of your paternal grandparents?

....

¿What were the names of your maternal grandparents?

....

| Date: ..../.............../............ | Duration: .... |
| Start time: .... | End time: .... |

Answer the questions:

¿Where did you study?

....

¿What year did you get married?

....

¿Who did you marry?

....

¿How many children do you have?

....

Write their names:

....

....

¿How many grandchildren do you have?

....

Date: ..../ ..../ .... Duration: ....

Start time: .... End time: ....

Pay close attention to the picture below. Write the names of eight (8) objects that you see in the image:

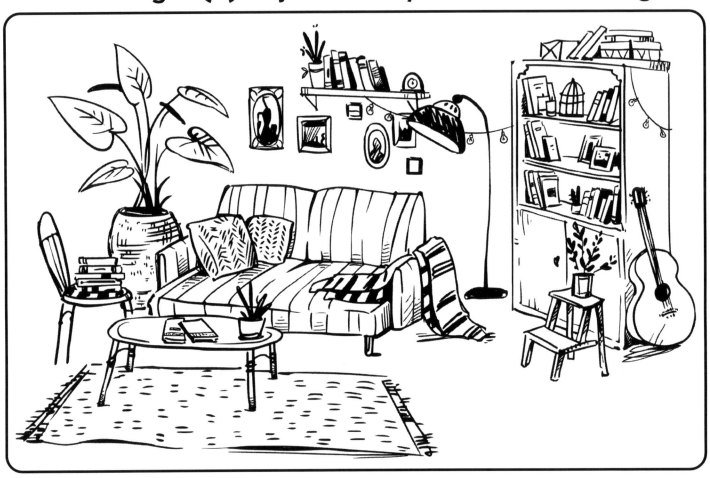

....

....

....

....

Date: ..../.............../..............	Duration: ....
Start time:	End time: ....

¿How many figures are there of each cat? Write down the number in each box:

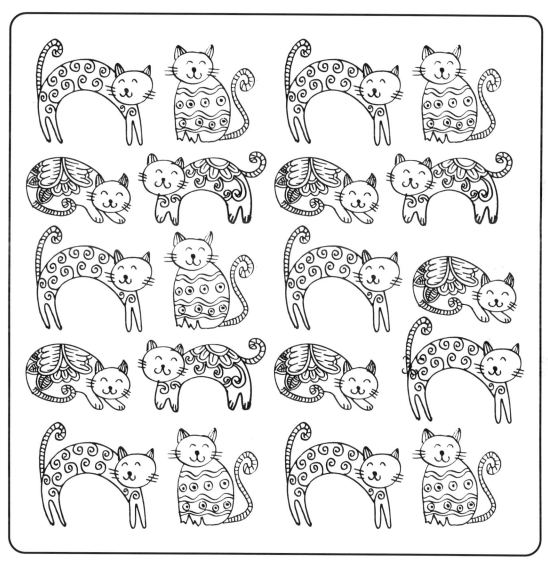

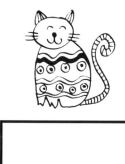
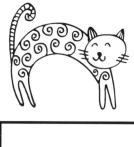
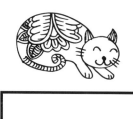
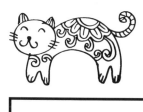

Cognitive Function: **PERCEPTION**

Date: ..../ ..../ ....   Duration: ....

Start time: ....   End time: ....

Draw a line to match the image with its respective silhouette:

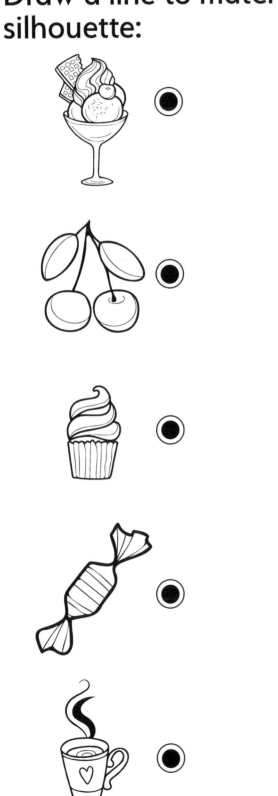
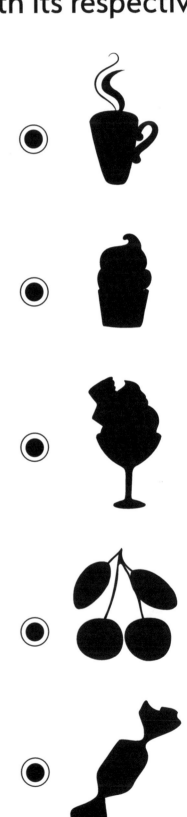

Date: ..../.............../............. Duration: ....

Start time: .... End time: ....

Arrange the sequence in each row and write the matching number in each box:

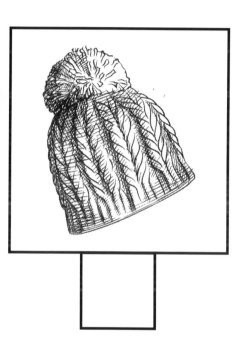

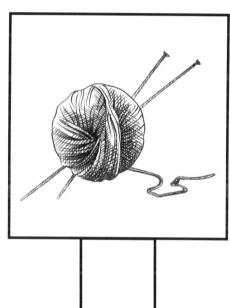

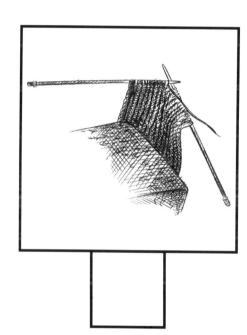

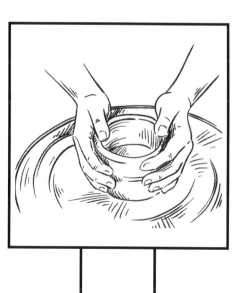

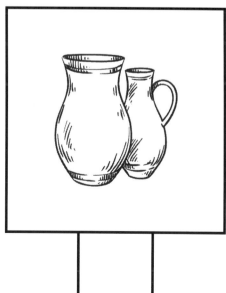

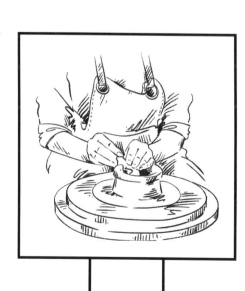

Date: ..../.............../............   Duration: ....

Start time: ....   End time: ....

Connect the dots following the sequence of numbers. Write the name of the musical instrument on the dotted line, and then color the picture.

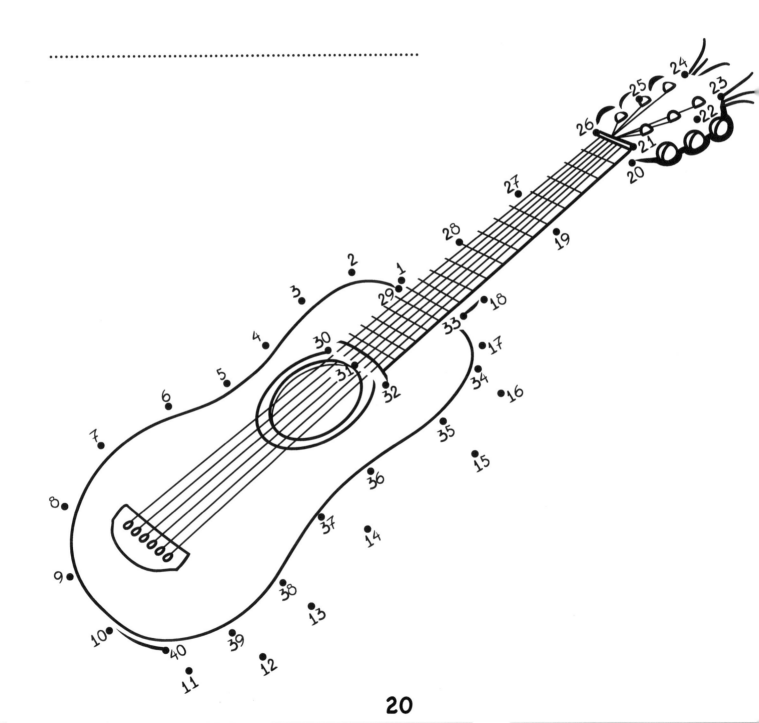

20

Date: ..../............../...............	Duration: ....
Start time:	End time: ....

Under each image, write the number that corresponds to it:

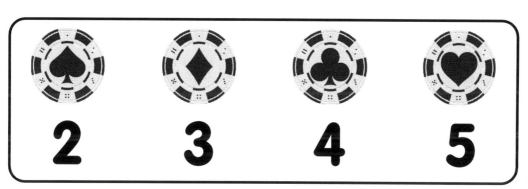

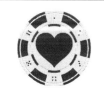

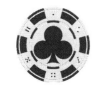

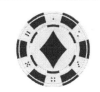

Circle the smallest number in each row:

9	4	7	1	8	3	6
10	6	9	11	8	7	12
11	9	13	8	14	12	16
5	8	7	9	12	3	11
12	10	11	14	9	17	14
19	12	4	8	11	9	7

Date: ..../ ..../ .... Duration: ....

Start time: .... End time: ....

Draw a line to connect each fruit's name with its corresponding image:

banana ◉ 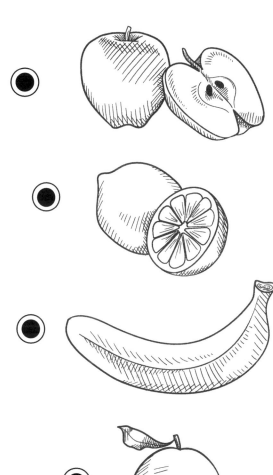 ◉

pineapple ◉ ◉

lemon ◉ ◉

apple ◉ ◉

orange ◉ 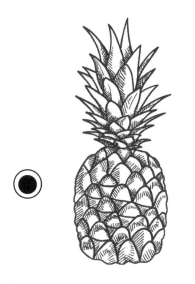 ◉

Date: ..../.............../...............   Duration: ....

Start time: ....   End time: ....

Write the letter A inside the figure ☐ and the letter B inside the figure ◌ :

Date: ..../.............../...............   Duration: ....

Start time: ....   End time: ....

Complete the drawing according to the figure in the box and then color the image:

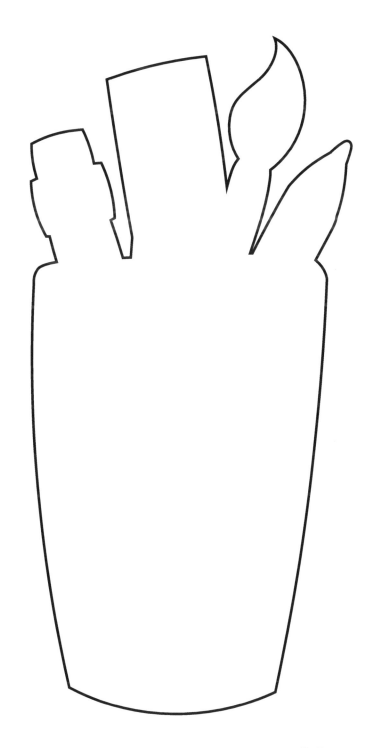

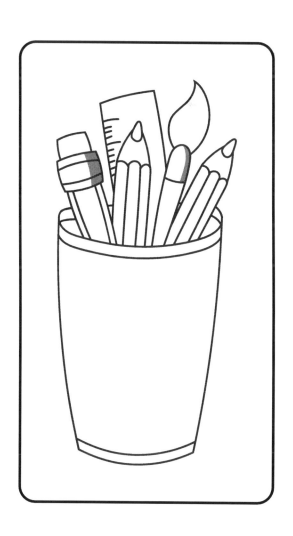

Date: ..../.............../...............   Duration: ....

Start time: ....   End time: ....

Mark with an **X** as many figures as the number that appears at the beginning of the row:

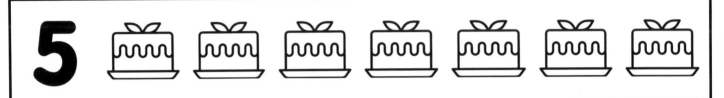

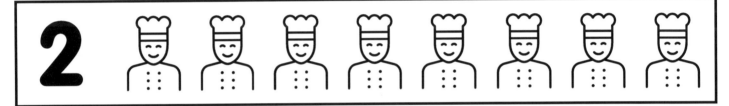

Date: ..../.............../.............   Duration: ....

Start time: ....   End time: ....

Look at the picture of the animal for 2 minutes, then go to the next page:

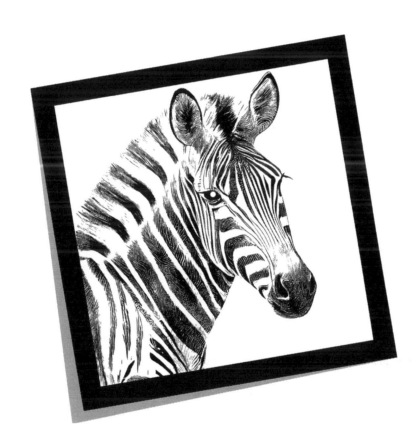

Cognitive Function: MEMORY

Mark with an **X** the image of the animal you saw on the previous page:

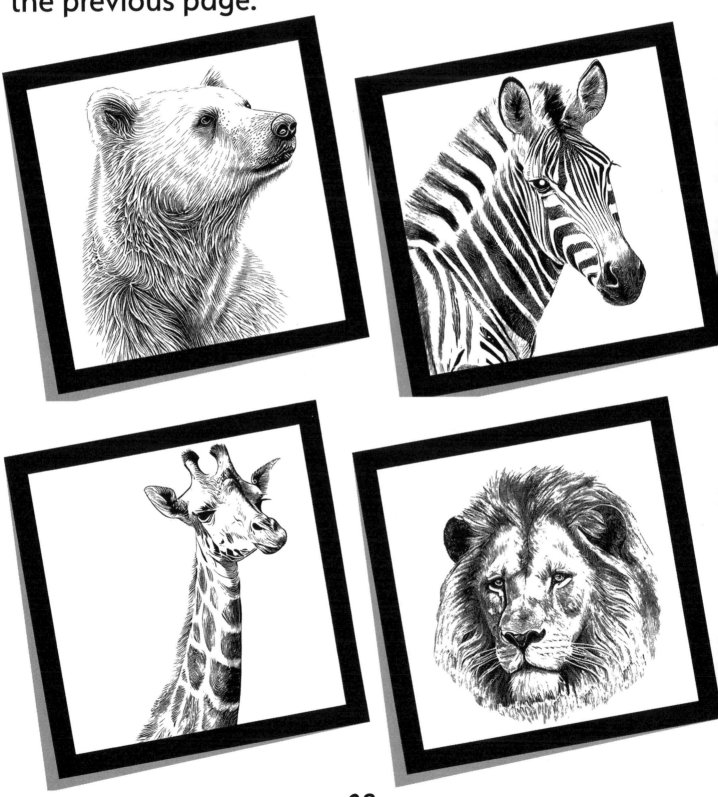

Date: ..../............/............   Duration: ....

Start time: ....   End time: ....

Write the largest number in each empty box, regardless of how big or small it looks:

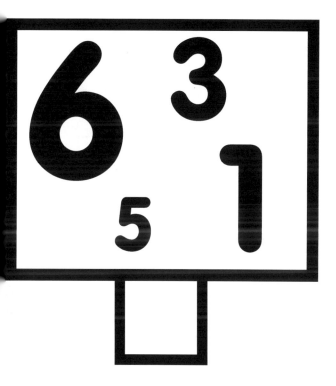

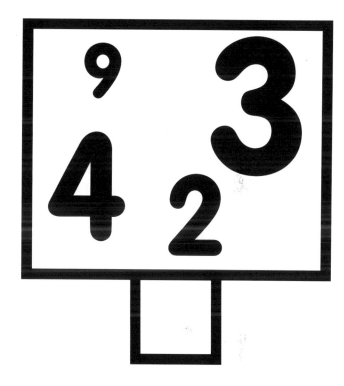

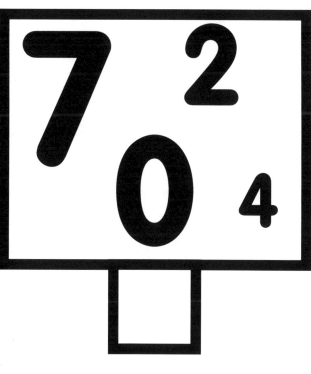

Date: ..../ ..../ ....

Duration: ....

Start time: ....

End time: ....

Put an **X** on the figure that repeats in each row:

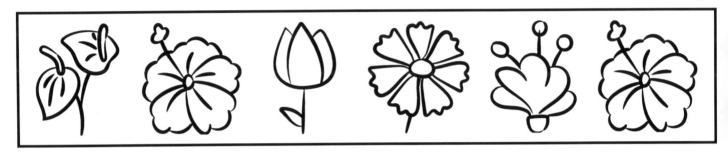

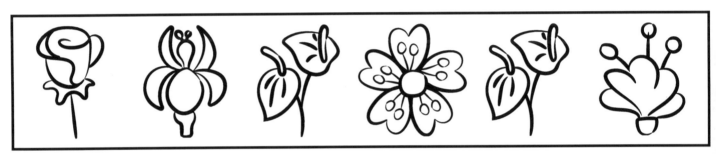

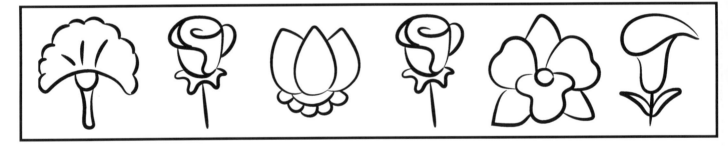

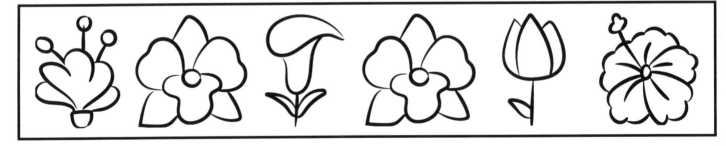

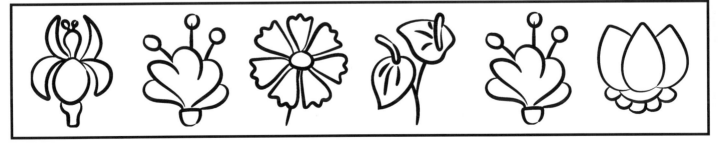

Date: ..../.............../............

Duration: ....

Start time: ....

End time: ....

Complete the word search:

- memory
- activity
- sleep
- healthy
- exercise
- live
- joy
- love
- autonomy

↓

→

X	H	E	A	L	T	H	Y	L	E
A	L	C	C	P	Ñ	K	P	Z	X
U	K	S	T	I	J	L	O	V	E
T	G	I	I	F	R	I	T	O	R
O	H	W	V	D	A	V	K	B	C
N	J	I	I	Q	U	E	J	V	I
O	T	D	T	N	S	X	L	R	S
M	Y	J	Y	J	O	Y	T	D	E
Y	X	D	S	X	S	L	E	E	P
R	T	M	E	M	O	R	Y	R	J

Date: ..../............../..............

Duration: ....

Start time: ....

End time: ....

Complete the sequence by adding the number above the arrow:

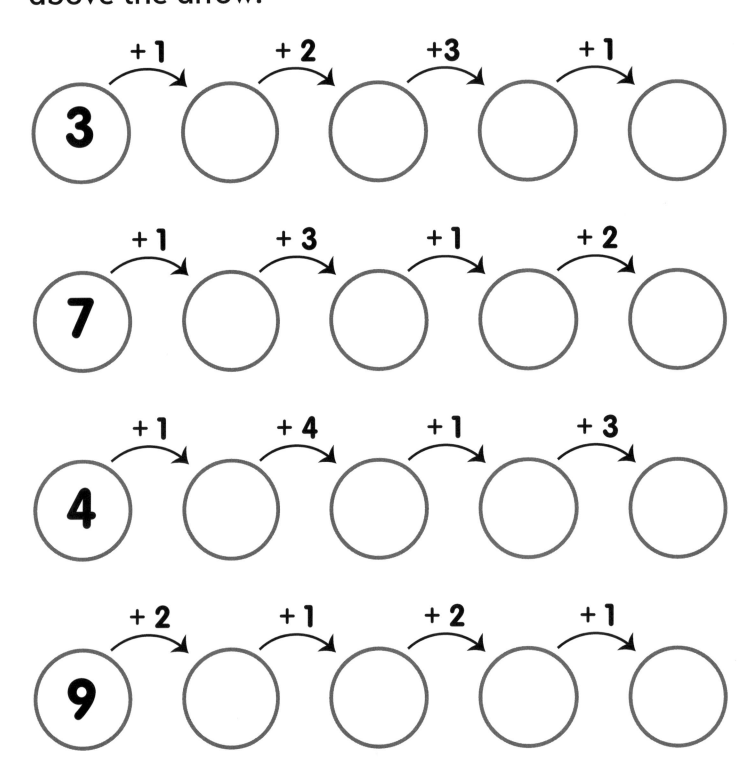

Date: ..../ ..../	Duration: ....
Start time:	End time: ....

In the image, mark with an **X** the objects mentioned in the list:

- chair
- pear
- candle
- table
- glass of wine
- books

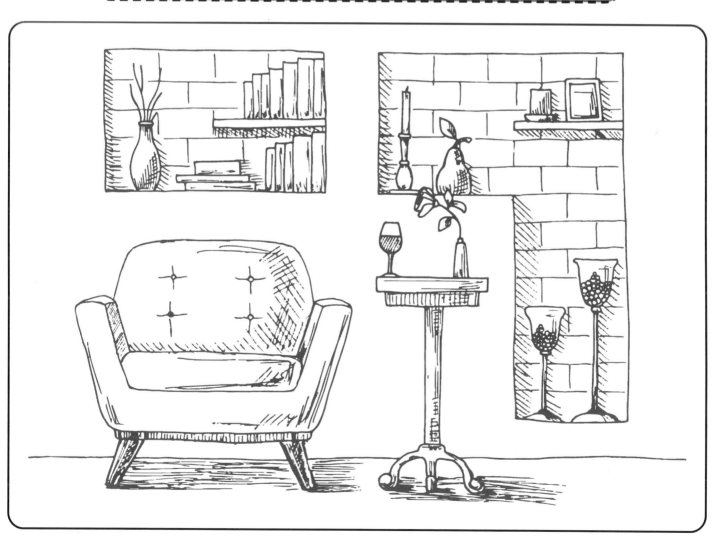

Date: ..../ ..../ ....   Duration: ....

Start time: ....   End time: ....

Read Aesop's fable and underline the letters **a**:

There was once a countryman who possessed the most wonderful goose you can imagine, for every day when he visited the nest, the goose had laid a beautiful, glittering, golden egg.

The countryman took the eggs to the market and soon began to get rich. But it was not long before he grew impatient with the goose because she gave him only a single golden egg a day. He was not getting rich fast enough.

Then one day, after he had finished counting his money, the idea came to him that he could get all the golden eggs at once by killing the goose and cutting it open. But when the deed was done, not a single golden egg did he find, and his precious goose was dead.

Count all the a's and then write the result number in the box.

Date: ..../.............../.............

Duration: ....

Start time: ....

End time: ....

Answer the following from the previous reading. You can reread the fable if you need to:

¿What is the title of the fable?

1 The Ants and the Grasshopper

2 The Goose & the Golden Egg

3 The Wolf and the Shepherd

¿What animal does the countryman have?

....

¿What was the material that was made of the goose's eggs?

....

¿What happened to the goose?

....

Date: ..../.............../.............

Duration: ....

Start time: ....

End time: ....

Connect the dots following the sequence of numbers. On the dotted line, write the name of the animal and then color the figure:

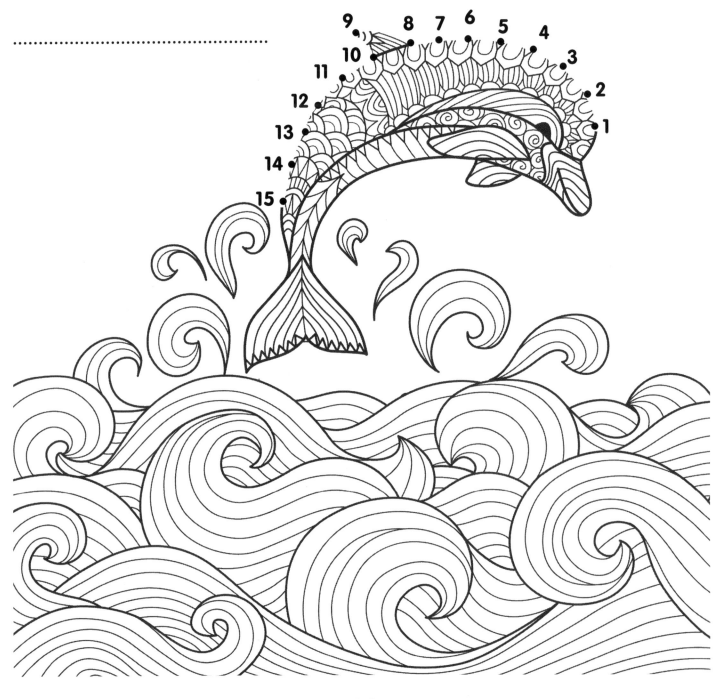

....

Date: ..../............../..............   Duration: ....

Start time: ....   End time: ....

Look at the following chair for 1 minute. Then turn to the next page.

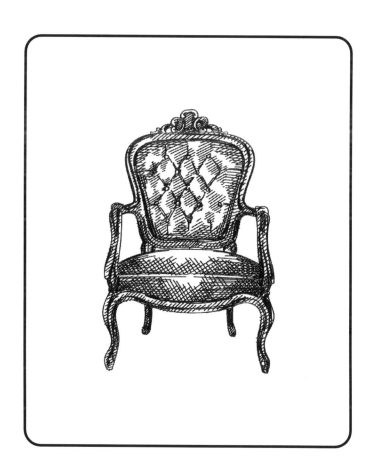

Date: ..../.............../............   Duration: ....

Start time: ....   End time: ....

Mark with an **X** the chair you saw on the previous page:

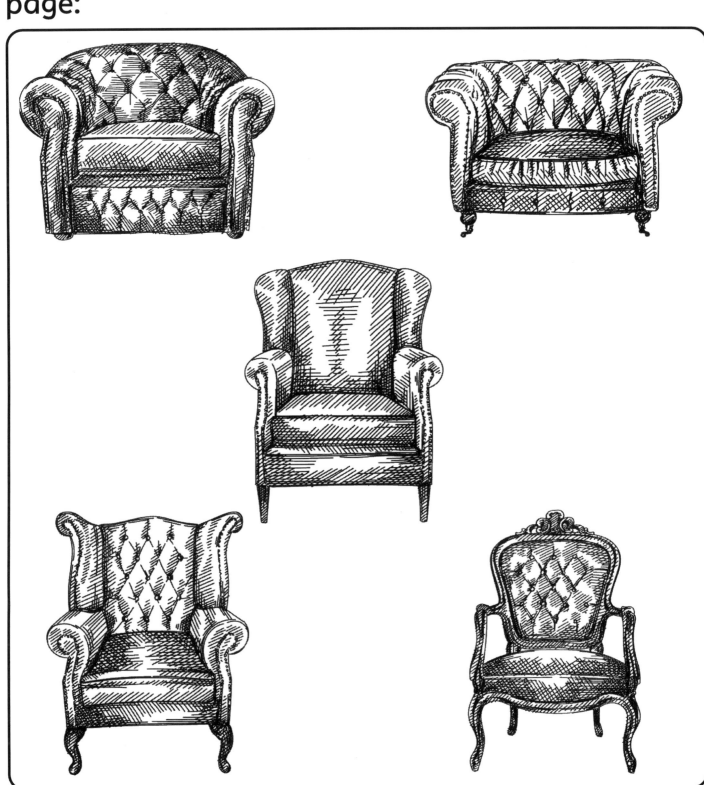

Date: ..../.............../.............

Duration: ....

Start time: ....

End time: ....

Mark with an **X** the silhouettes of the birds that are facing right and circle the silhouettes that are facing left:

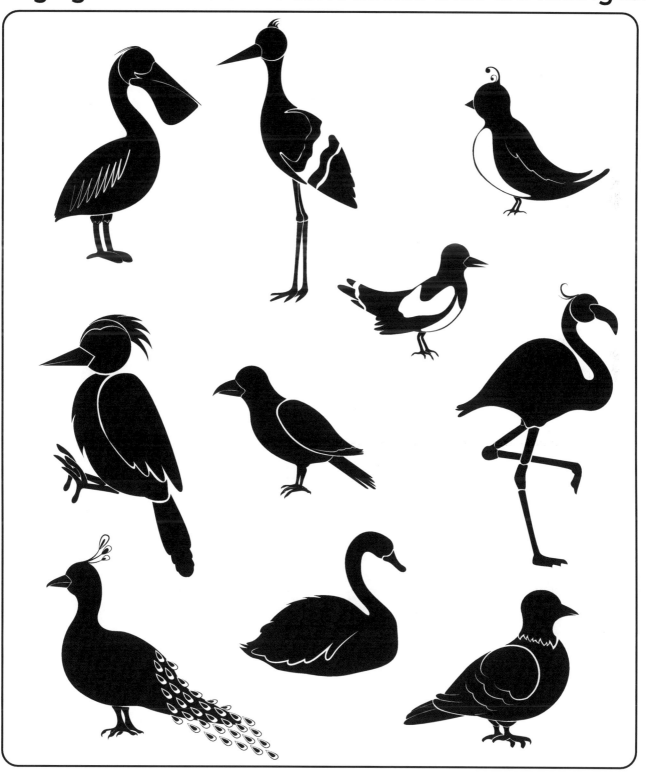

Date: ..../ ..../ ....

Duration: ....

Start time: ....

End time: ....

Search for the hidden numbers in the grid:

- 3516
- 8321
- 9287
- 2840
- 1765
- 5687
- 9248
- 7903
- 7534

8	5	2	8	4	0	2	4	5	0
1	6	5	4	7	8	4	6	1	7
7	7	5	2	4	3	1	8	5	6
5	1	3	7	5	2	7	3	6	5
3	7	5	0	6	1	6	8	8	5
4	0	3	5	1	6	5	0	7	4
1	4	8	9	4	5	6	0	2	8
1	3	9	0	2	6	4	1	9	8
9	2	4	8	4	9	2	8	7	2
7	4	7	9	0	3	1	0	2	6

Date: ..../ ..../ ....

Duration: ....

Start time: ....

End time: ....

Look at the image of each appliance and fill in the missing letters to complete the name:

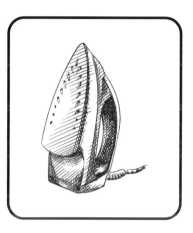

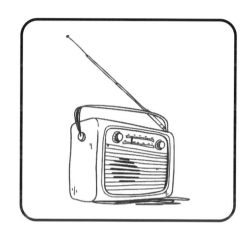

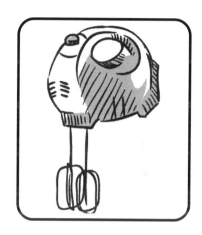

i _ o _

r _ _ i _

m _ x _ _

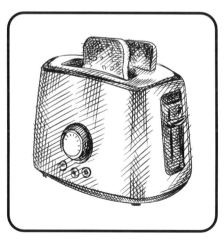

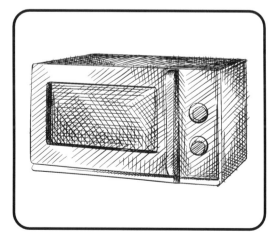

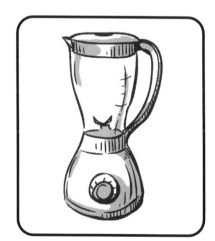

t _ a _ _ e _

m _ c _ _ w _ _ e

b _ e _ _ _ _

Date: ..../.............../...........

Duration: ....

Start time: ....

End time: ....

Mark with an **X** the letters you find:

K	8	L	M	3
2	J	G	1	H
F	B	9	P	5
3	T	C	4	L
R	5	B	P	2
E	1	Z	7	U

Date: ..../.............../..............   Duration: ....

Start time: ....   End time: ....

Write the respective profession below each figure:

doctor, singer, fireman, scientist,
artist, chef, athlete, policeman, mechanic

....

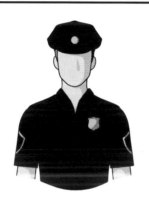

....

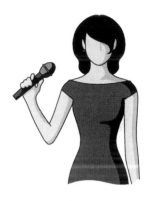

....

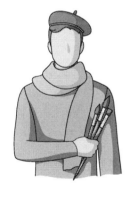

....

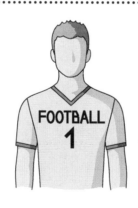

....

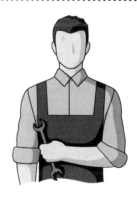

....

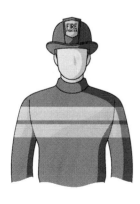

....

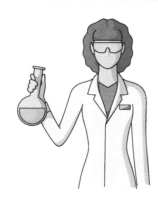

....

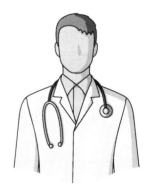

....

Date: ..../.............../............   Duration: ....

Start time: ....   End time: ....

You are going on a trip, where would you go? Next, list the names of ten items you would pack in your suitcase:

Place: ....

Items: ....

....

....

....

....

....

....

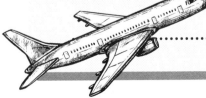

Date: ..../ .... / ....

Duration: ....

Start time: ....

End time: ....

Help the teapot reach the teacup by following the consecutive numbers. Mark each number with an **X**:

56	22	47	50	71	29	74
30	68	42	77	25	51	82
▶1	2	3	4	59	80	36
23	54	39	65	33	73	5	64	28	76

23	54	39	65	33	73	5	64	28	76
37	11	10	9	8	7	6	55	31	79
80	12	43	60	27	67	48	24	75	61
44	13	38	53	72	34	40	63	58	26
62	14	15	16	52	45	81			
32	57	70	17	18	78	49			
41	66	35	46	19	20	21▶			

Date: ..../............../..............   Duration: ....

Start time: ....   End time: ....

Write the names of ten (10) objects you see in the image:

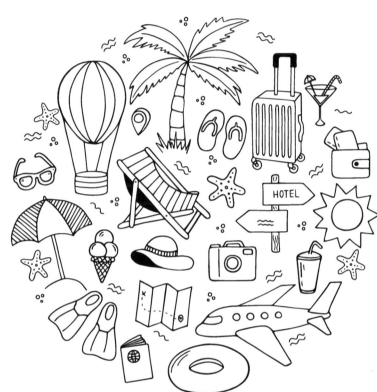

....

....

....

....

Date: ..../.............../...............   Duration: ....

Start time: ....   End time: ....

Memorize the images, their names, and their locations for 2 minutes. Then turn to the next page.

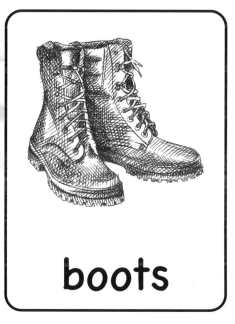

boots

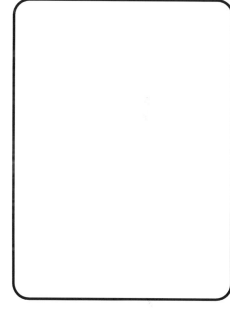

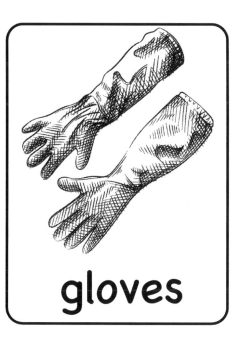

gloves

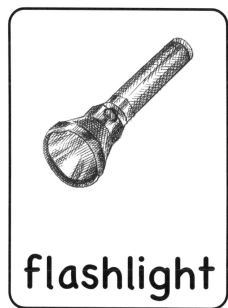

flashlight

Date: ..../............../..............   Duration: ....

Start time: ....   End time: ....

Write the name of each object on the dotted line in the box where it was placed on the previous page:

....

....

| Date: ..../ .... / .... | Duration: .... |
| Start time: .... | End time: .... |

Mark with an **X** the silhouette of the geometric figure that corresponds to the box on the left:

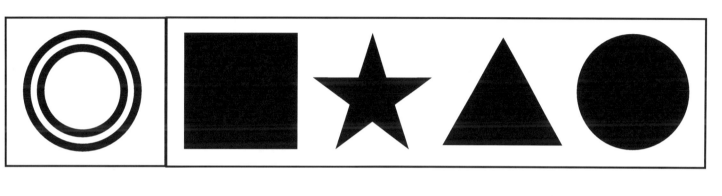

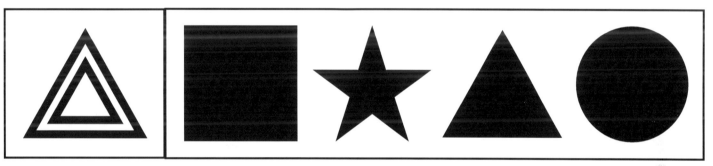

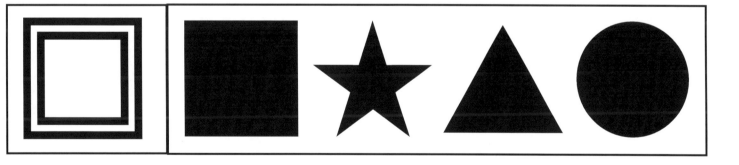

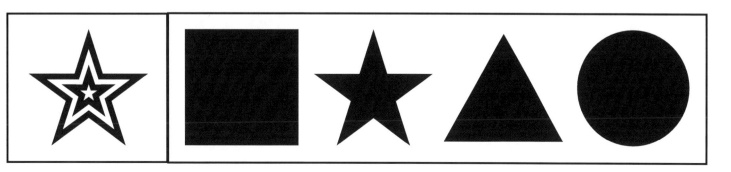

Cognitive Function: MATH

| Date: ...../...../..... | Duration: .... |
| Start time: .... | End time: .... |

Add the numbers on the dice in each box and write the total inside the circle:

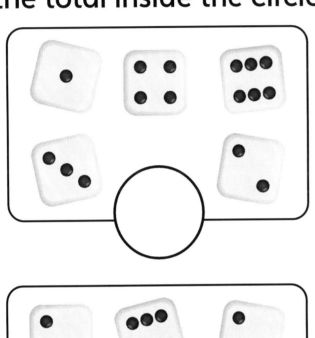

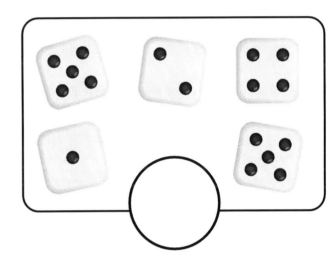

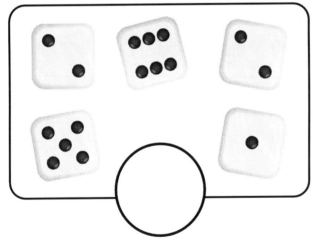

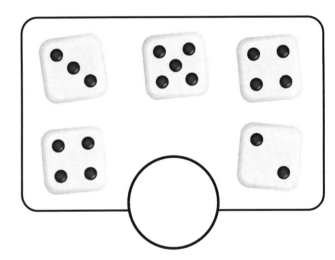

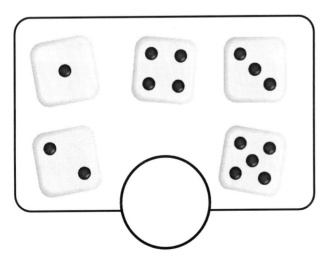

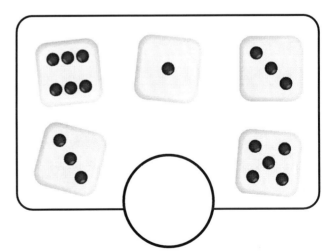

Date: ..../.............../............. Duration: ....

Start time: .... End time: ....

Find and mark with an **X** the image of the clock that does NOT have a pair:

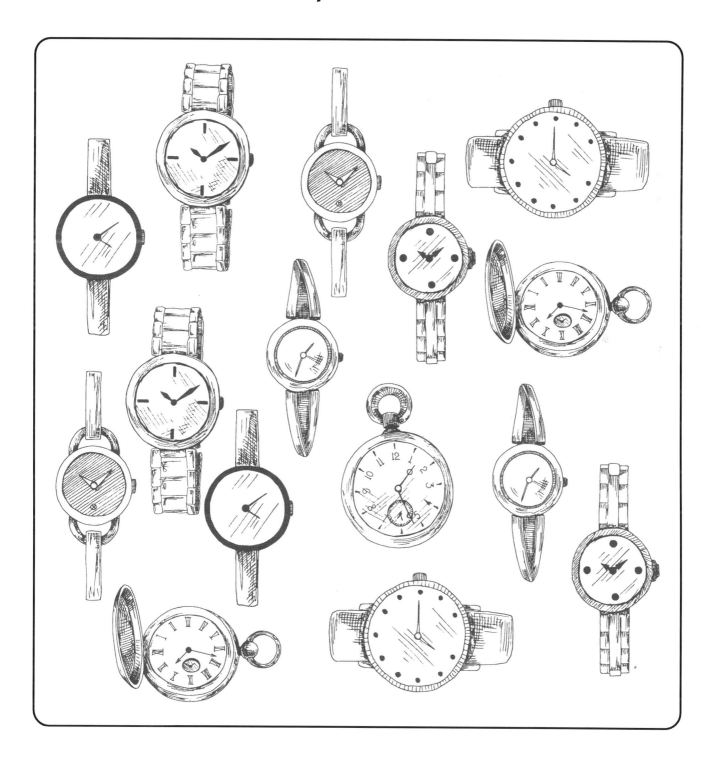

Connect the dots to form the 2 parts of the proverb:

No pain ◉

Don't judge ◉

Not gain ◉

Out of sight ◉

Every dog ◉

Better safe ◉

Rome was not built ◉

◉ than sorry

◉ has its day

◉ no gain

◉ by its cover

◉ in one day

◉ without pain

◉ out of mind

Cognitive Function: **LANGUAGE**

Date: ..../................/...............	Duration: ....
Start time:	End time: ....

Write six (6) proverbs different from those mentioned on the previous page:

1 ....
....

2 ....
....

3 ....
....

4 ....
....

5 ....
....

6 ....
....

Date: ..../............../..............   Duration: ....

Start time: ....   End time: ....

Solve the Sudoku. Fill the empty boxes with numbers from 1 to 6. Each row, column, and 2x3 box must include the numbers 1 to 6 without repeating:

2		1	4	5	6
6	4		2		
1	2	4		6	
	5		1	4	2
	1	3	6	2	4
4		2		1	3

Date: ..../.............../.............

Duration: ....

Start time: ....

End time: ....

Mark with an **X** the missing puzzle piece to complete the picture:

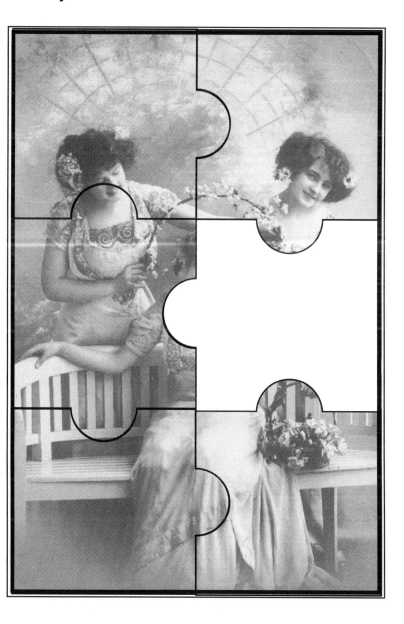
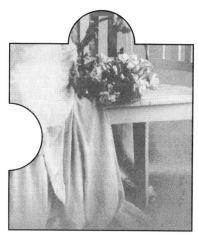
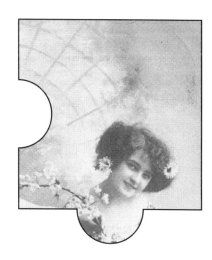
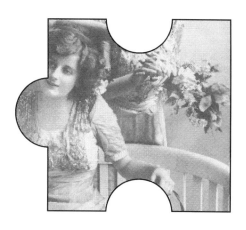

Date: ..../.............../............

Duration: ....

Start time: ....

End time: ....

In front of each image, write the activity that each person is doing:

....

....

....

....

....

....

....

....

Date: ..../.............../............   Duration: ....

Start time: ....   End time: ....

Complete the crossword puzzle:

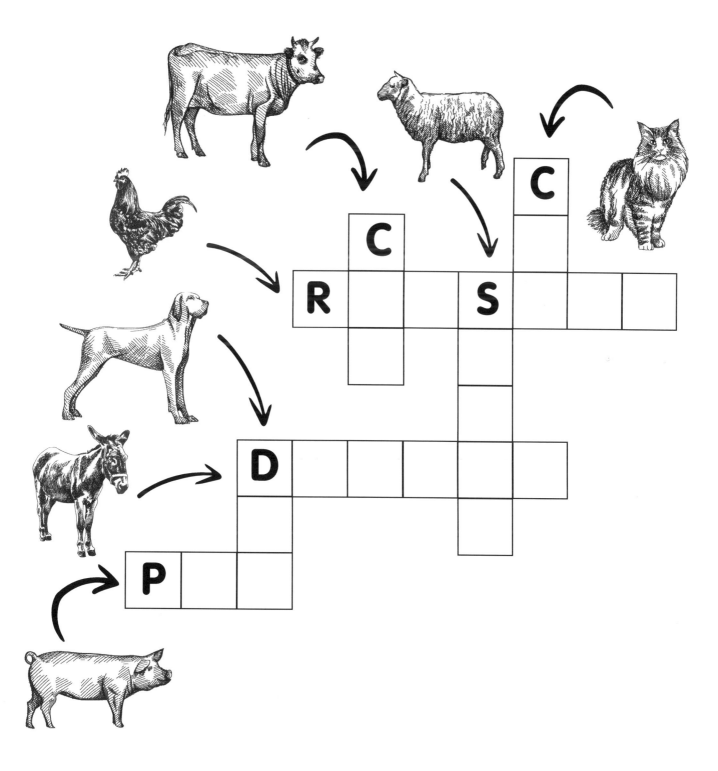

Date: ..../.............../...............

Duration: ....

Start time: ....

End time: ....

In each box, draw the missing half of the picture:

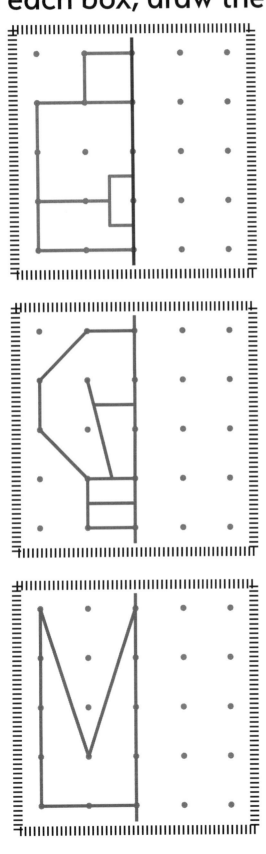
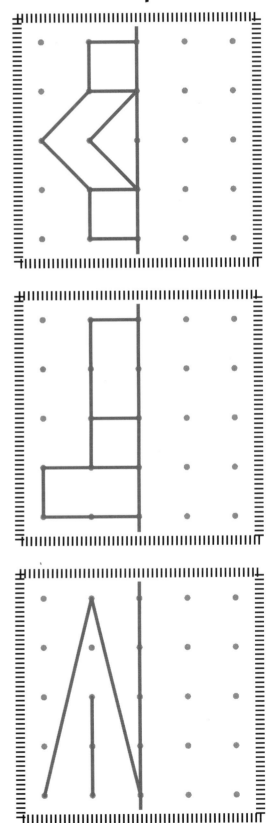

Date: ..../.............../..............   Duration: ....

Start time: ....   End time: ....

Look at the following items used to make cookies. Memorize them. Then go to the next page.

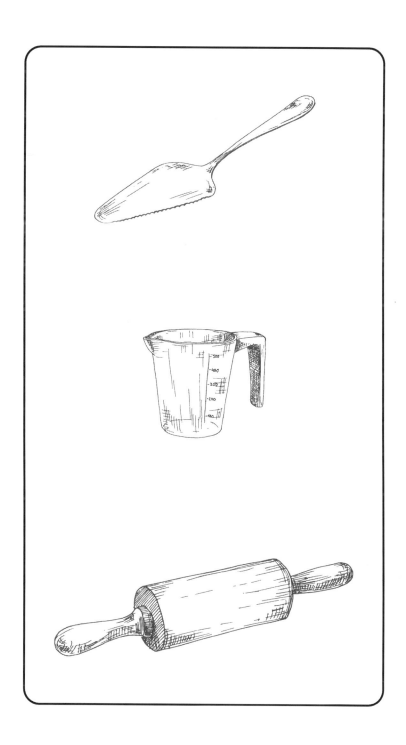

| Date: ..../.............../............. | Duration: .... |
| Start time: .... | End time: .... |

Mark with an X the 3 (three) objects you memorized from the previous page:

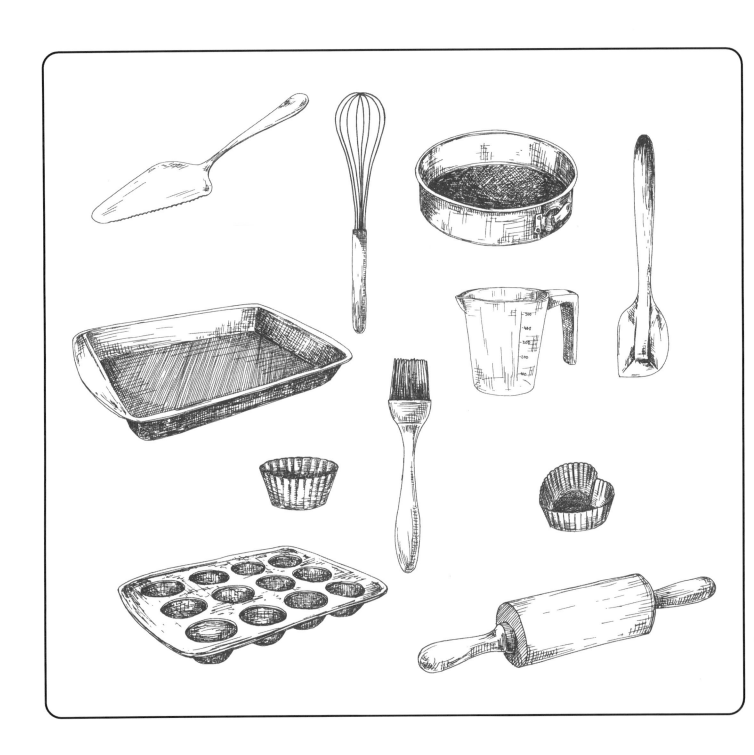

Date: ..../ ..../ ....   Duration: ....

Start time: ....   End time: ....

Mark with an **X** the even numbers and circle the odd numbers:

17	1	50	12	29	21	33	14
64	39	60	55	42	48	7	51
4	61	25	15	3	20	45	38
11	31	8	41	24	37	30	56
22	36	2	54	9	49	26	62
63	32	47	44	16	43	59	10
40	19	52	57	35	27	5	58
6	46	28	23	34	13	53	18

Date: ..../.............../.............

Duration: ....

Start time: ....

End time: ....

Write the missing numbers:

1				5					10
	12			15		17	18		
21			24		26			29	
	32			35					40
		43			46		48		
	52			55				59	
		63			66		68		70
71				75				79	
	82		84			87			90
91		93			96			99	

Date: ..../............../............

Duration: ....

Start time: ....

End time: ....

Mark with an **X** the object that does NOT belong to the group:

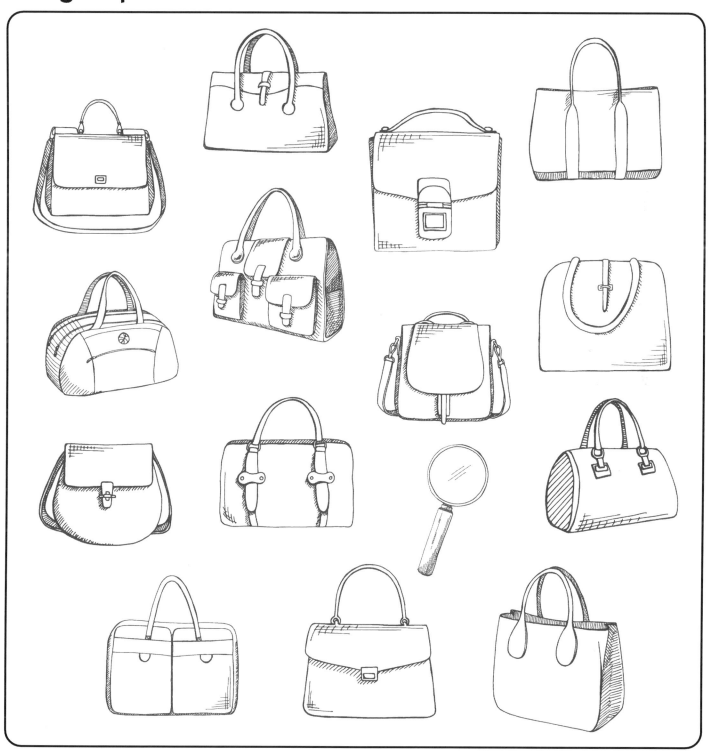

Date: ..../ ..../ ....   Duration: ....

Start time: ....   End time: ....

Write on the lines the phrase you see on the fence:

Live your life and forget your age

....

....

....

....

Date: ..../.............../.............   Duration: ....

Start time: ....   End time: ....

Write in each blank box the missing number (it is the result of subtracting the two numbers):

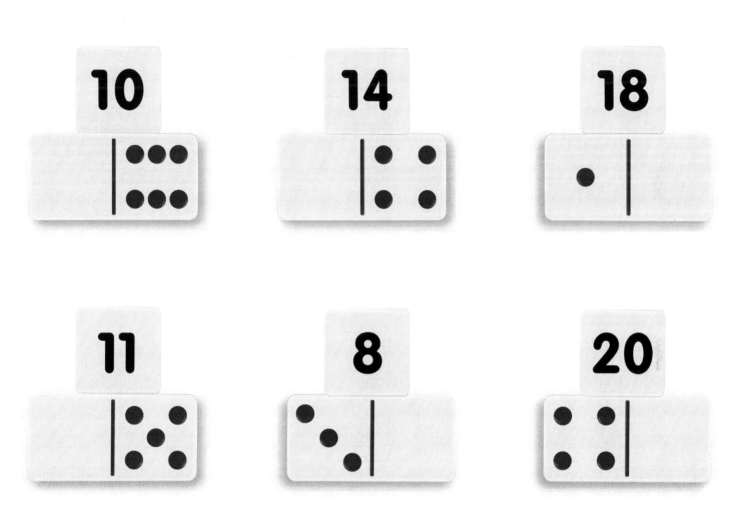

Date: ..../.............../.............   Duration: ....

Start time: ....   End time: ....

Color the image and then mention the name of three (3) objects:

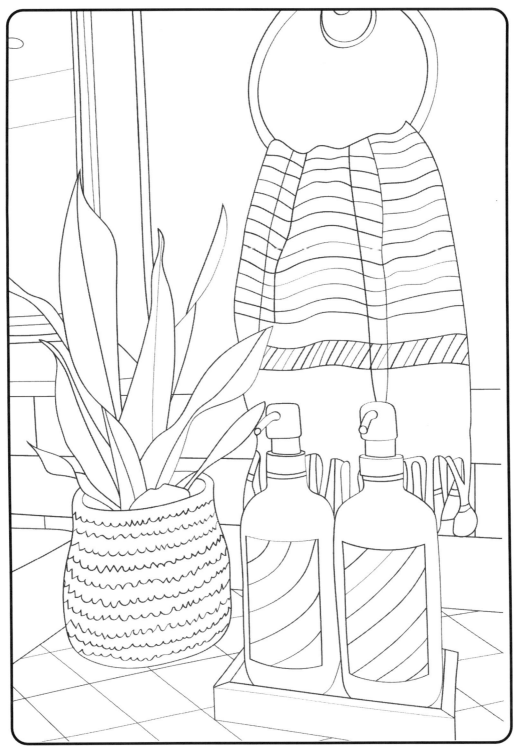

Date: ..../ ..../ ....   Duration: ....

Start time: ....   End time: ....

According to the details provided in the box, write below each image what it is used for:

> to display the time - to carry money -
> for watering plants - to cook food -
> to prevent theft - to produce light

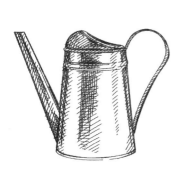 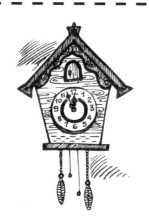 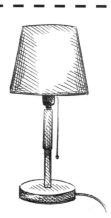

....

....

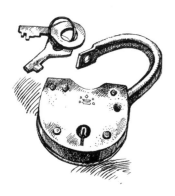 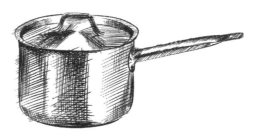 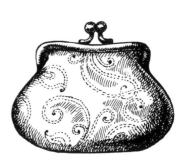

....

....

Cognitive Function: **PERCEPTION**

Date: ..../.............../.............

Start time: ....

Duration: ....

End time: ....

Draw a line to match the images of shoes that are the same:

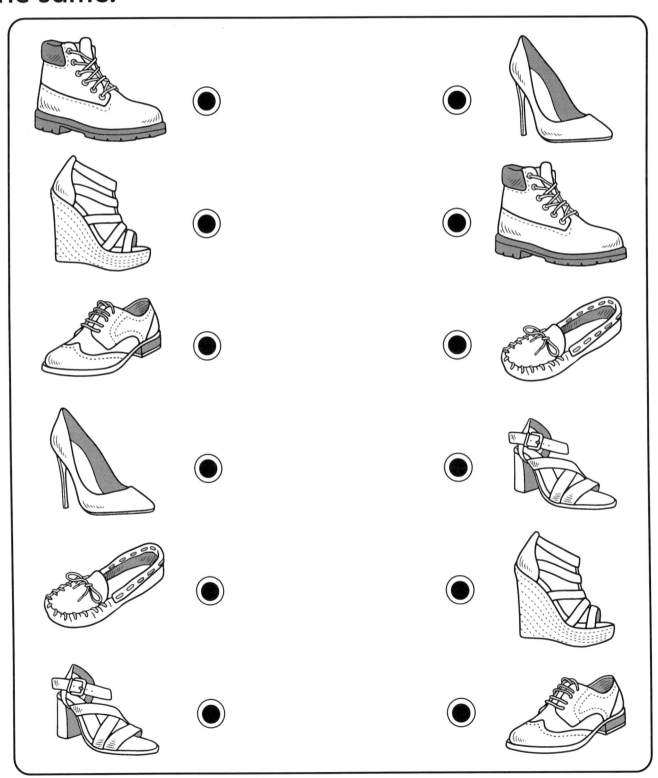

Cognitive Function: **MEMORY**

Pay close attention to the following picture and try to memorize it. Say out loud the objects you see. Then go to the next page.

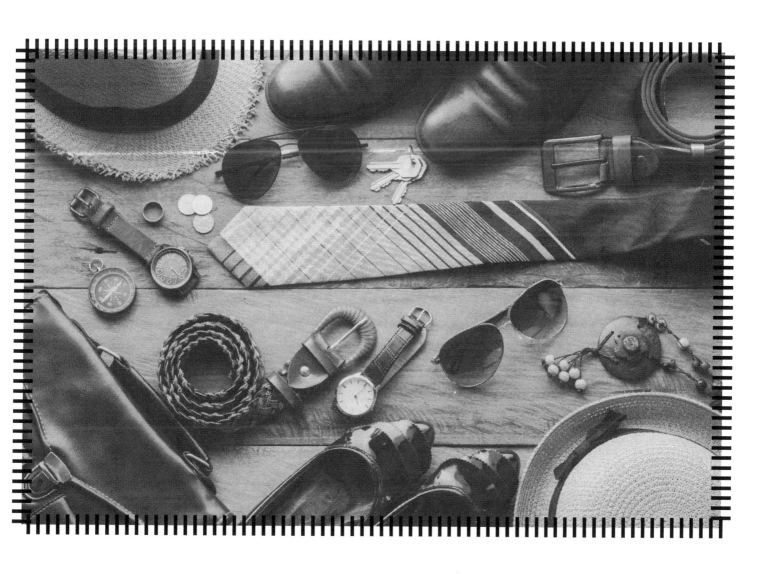

69

Cognitive Function: MEMORY

| Date: ..../ ..../ .... | Duration: .... |
| Start time: .... | End time: .... |

From the image you saw on the previous page, write the name of the largest number of objects you remember:

◉

....

◉

....

◉

....

◉

....

◉

....

◉

....

◉

....

◉

....

Date: ..../............./.............	Duration: ....
Start time:	End time: ....

Write the time shown below each clock:

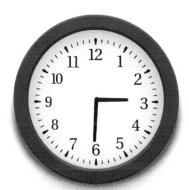

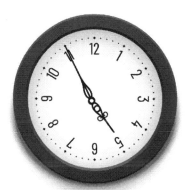

....

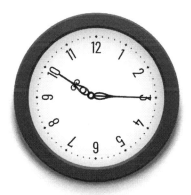

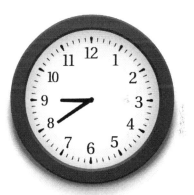

....

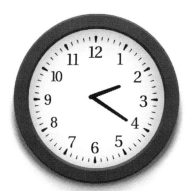

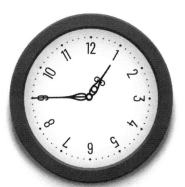

....

Date: ..../.............../............

Duration: ....

Start time: ....

End time: ....

Mark with an **X** the image that is the same size as the one in the box on the left:

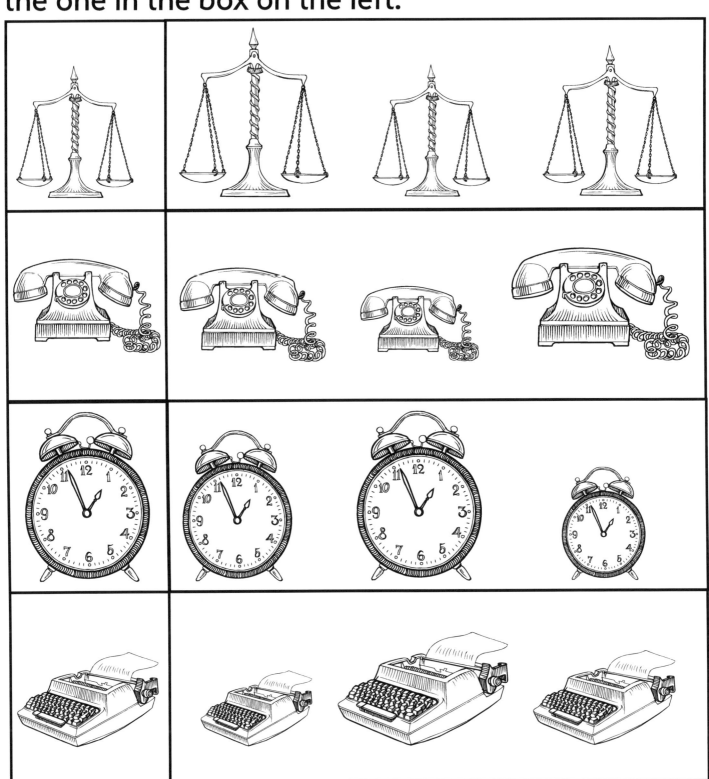

Draw the missing half of the picture:

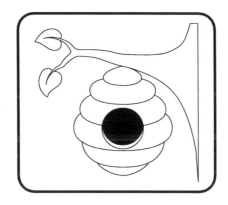

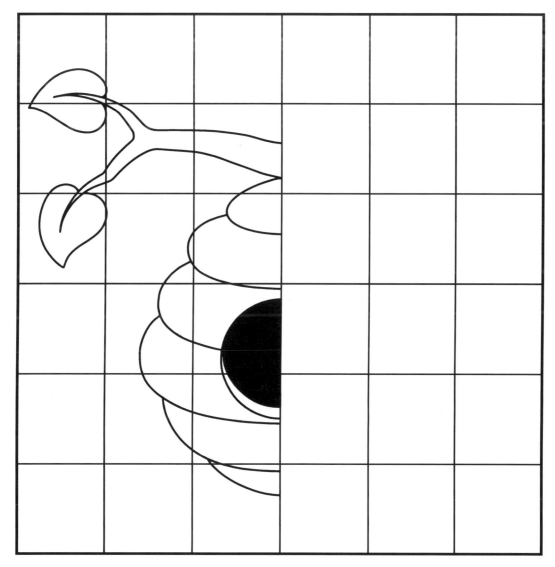

Date: ..../.............../.............

Duration: ....

Start time: ....

End time: ....

Complete the word search:

- joyful
- popular
- friends
- wishes
- celebration
- birthday
- presents
- guests
- party

B	I	R	T	H	D	A	Y	O	S	X	J
C	S	D	O	F	G	Y	P	M	N	L	O
E	Q	P	S	L	P	T	P	A	R	T	Y
L	S	O	U	Y	B	G	L	G	N	F	F
E	T	P	L	N	F	U	J	X	V	B	U
B	Q	U	F	R	I	E	N	D	S	P	L
R	V	L	R	X	E	S	H	Q	G	L	J
A	T	A	X	F	S	T	Q	Z	U	T	E
T	Q	R	H	Z	T	S	D	S	E	R	G
I	P	D	C	P	R	E	S	E	N	T	S
O	T	R	S	D	F	H	Q	P	T	Y	N
N	S	A	G	W	I	S	H	E	S	Q	P

In each row, follow the sequence and draw the respective geometric figure in the blank boxes:

Date: ..../.............../............

Duration: ....

Start time: ....

End time: ....

Solve the Sudoku. Fill the empty boxes with the numbers 1 through 9. Each row, column, and 3 x 3 box must contain the numbers 1 through 9:

6		5	3		2
3		1	6	5	4
5	6	3	2		1
2			5	6	
4	5	2		3	6
	3		4	2	

Mark with an **X** the figure equal to 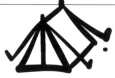 :

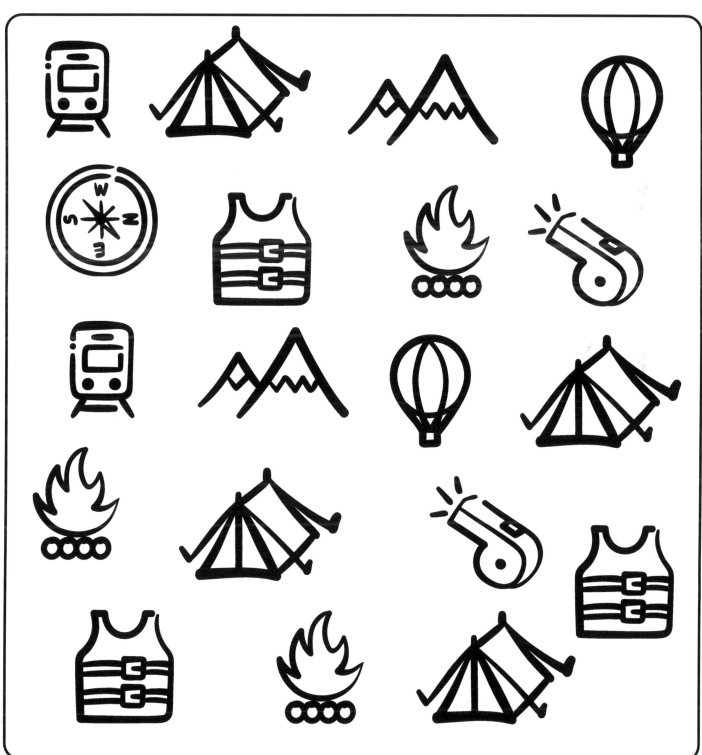

Date: ..../ ..../ ....   Duration: ....

Start time: ....   End time: ....

Below each image, write the name of the respective sensory organs:

smell - taste - sight - hearing

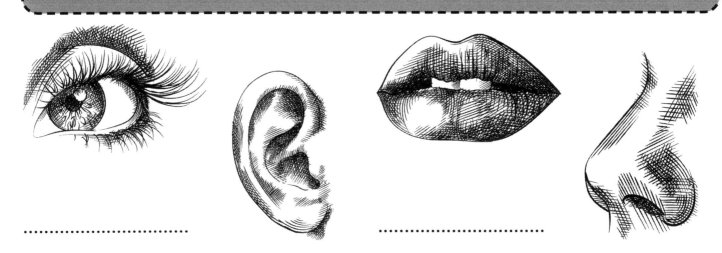

....

....

Answer the following questions:

- I can see with my ....
- I can hear with my ....
- I can eat with my ....
- I can smell with my ....

| Date: ..../.............../............ | Duration: .... |
| Start time: .... | End time: .... |

Look at the following objects and try to memorize them. Then go to the next page.

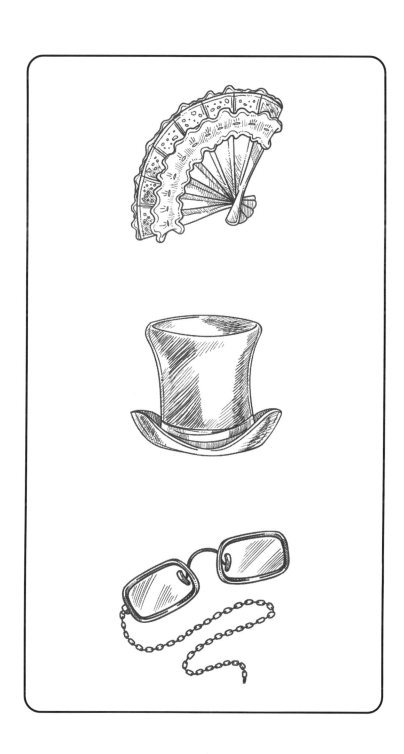

Cognitive Function: **MEMORY**

Date: ..../ ..../ .... Duration: ....

Start time: .... End time: ....

Mark with an **X** the 3 (three) objects that you memorized on the previous page:

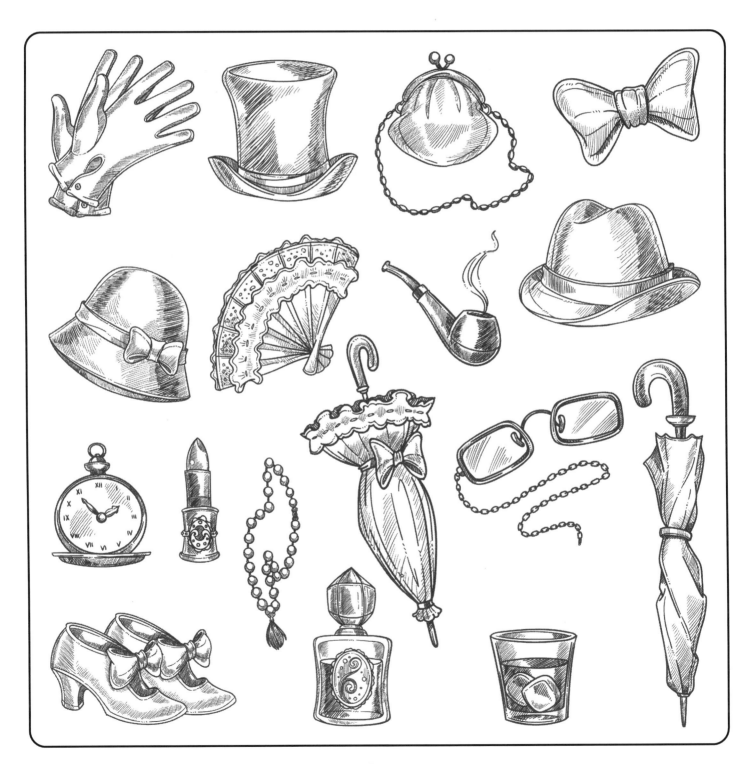

Cognitive Function: MATH

Mark with an **X** two numbers in each box to obtain the result indicated in the circle:

```
4 8 3
7 1 9  = 12
5 6 2
```

```
3 4 7
2 5 8  = 9
1 6 9
```

```
2 3 1
5 4 8  = 15
6 7 9
```

```
1 6 9
4 5 8  = 7
3 7 2
```

```
9 4 8
5 6 7  = 13
3 2 1
```

```
2 4 3
1 5 8  = 16
6 7 9
```

```
4 6 3
5 9 8  = 14
2 7 1
```

```
1 4 7
2 5 8  = 11
3 6 9
```

```
6 5 4
2 1 3  = 12
7 8 9
```

```
1 2 3
4 9 7  = 10
5 6 8
```

```
3 8 5
6 1 9  = 8
4 7 2
```

Date: ..../.............../.............   Duration: ....

Start time: ....   End time: ....

There are 5 (five) differences between the two pictures below. Can you find them?

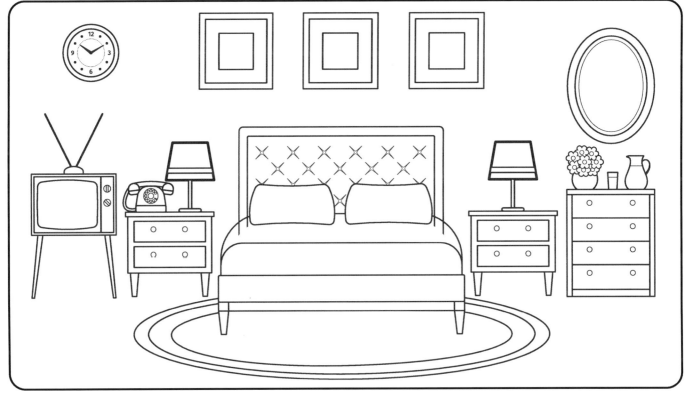

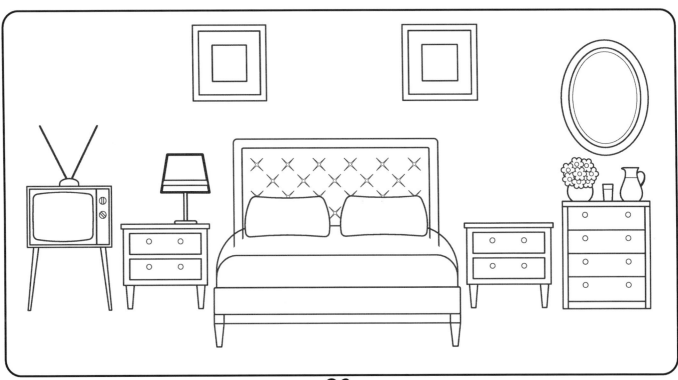

Date: ..../................/.............   Duration: ....

Start time: ....   End time: ....

Color the image:

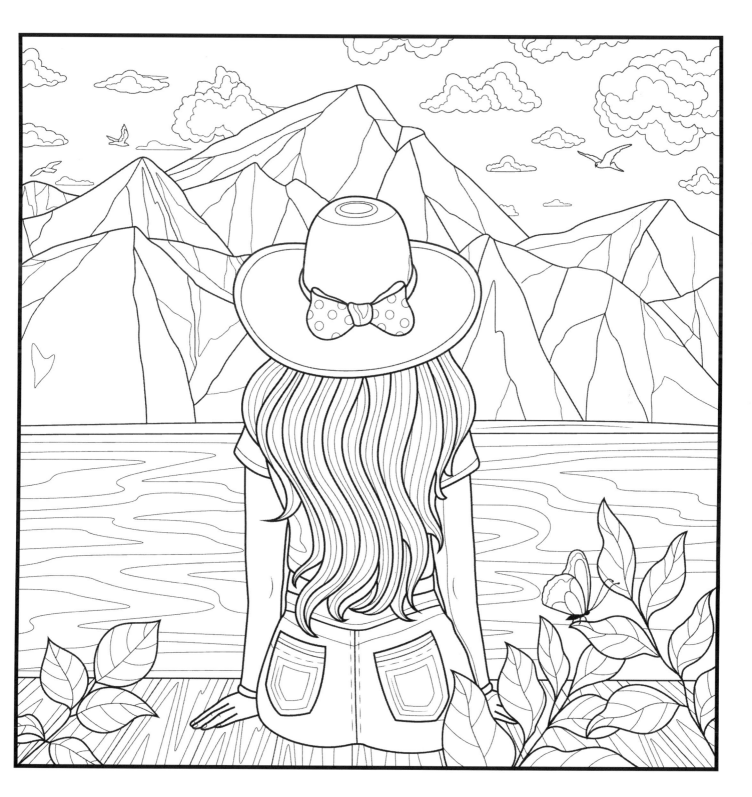

Date: ..../............../.............

Duration: ....

Start time: ....

End time: ....

Classify the words in the box in each box according to the respective category:

dolphin – white – cherry – lion – gray
cat – lemon – blue – dog – apple – bull
– black – coconut – green – grape

COLORS	FRUITS	ANIMALS
....	....	....
....	....	....
....	....	....
....	....	....
....	....	....

Date: ..../ ..../ ....

Duration: ....

Start time: ....

End time: ....

Complete the number search:

- 1037
- 3412
- 9708
- 9034
- 2268
- 6414
- 6512
- 9416
- 1941

↓

→

1	9	9	0	7	5	9	6	5	0
2	8	0	0	4	9	4	1	6	5
3	1	9	6	4	1	4	4	0	8
6	7	7	2	0	7	6	5	3	9
1	8	0	6	2	2	6	8	6	7
1	3	8	3	4	1	2	8	5	0
9	0	1	0	2	1	8	2	1	8
4	2	2	3	3	9	1	9	2	5
1	4	7	1	9	0	3	4	0	5
5	1	0	3	7	6	5	2	0	2

Date: ..../.............../............

Duration: ....

Start time: ....

End time: ....

Write on the line why the words are related:

flowers, days, clothes, months, colors
furniture, women's names, transportation

cat   dog   cow   animals ....

friday tuesday sunday.............................

skirt   shirt   pants ....

march may   april ....

green   blue   red ....

chair   bed   table ....

train   boat   plane ....

Lisa   Emily   Helen ....

daisy   rose   pons ....

Date: ..../ ..../ ....   Duration: ....

Start time: ....   End time: ....

Complete the words with the missing letter:

THE FOX & THE GRAPES -Aesop

A Fox _ne day spied a be_utiful bunch of ripe gr_pes hanging from a v_ne train_d along the br_nches of a tr_e. The gr_pes seemed read_ to burst with ju_ce, and the F_x's mouth wat_red as he gazed longingly at th_m.

The bunch hung from a h_gh branch, and the Fox h_d to jump for it. The f_rst time he j_mped he missed it by a l_ng way. So he walked off a sh_rt distance and to_k a running le_p at it, only to f_ll short once more. Ag_in and again he tried, but in va_n.

Now he s_t down and looked at the grapes in disg_st.

"What a f_ol I am," he said. "H_re I am wearing m_self out to get a bunch of s_ur grapes th_t are not worth g_ping for."

And off he w_lked ver_, very scornfully.

Date: ..../.............../.............   Duration: ....

Start time: ....   End time: ....

Write the name of 5 objects or words according to the instructions in each box:

CITIES

....

....

....

....

....

HOME APPLIANCES

....

....

....

....

....

FOOD

....

....

....

....

....

CLEANING ITEMS

....

....

....

....

....

Date: ..../............../..............

Duration: ....

Start time: ....

End time: ....

Draw a line to connect the two images and make the complete object:

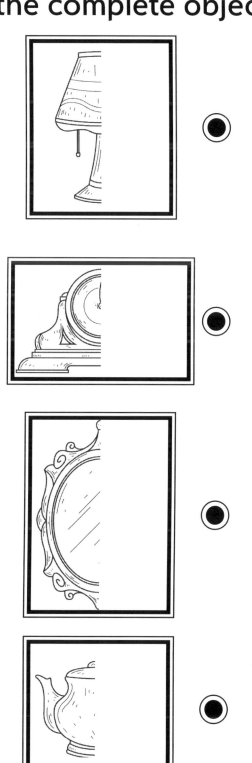
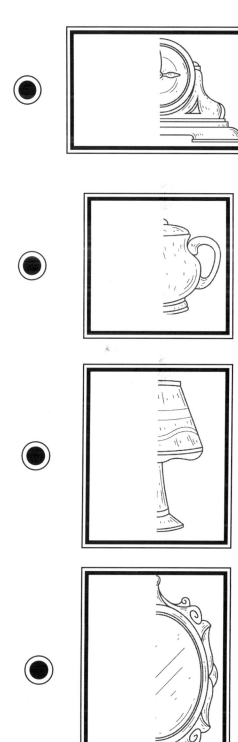

Cognitive Function: ORIENTATION

In each circle below the letters, write the correct letter in the right direction:

Date: ..../.............../.............   Duration: ....

Start time: ....   End time: ....

Write a word that means the same thing (synonym):

start – roof – sheet – end – soft
costly – annually – broad – large

yearly ....

ceiling ....

tender ....

expensive ....

big ....

page ....

begin ....

wide ....

finish ....

Date: ..../.............../.............   Duration: ....

Start time: ....   End time: ....

Above the line, write the letter corresponding to each box according to the instructions. Form the word:

	A	B	C	D
1	n	e	b	d
2	r	t	g	u
3	f	a	p	k
4	r	n	h	t

....

C2	A4	B1	B3	D4

Answer the questions:

What color is a strawberry?

....

Where do children study?

....

How many months are there in a year?

....

What foods come from cows?

....

Which utensil do you use to eat soup?

....

What is wine made of?

....

Date: ..../.............../........... Duration: ....

Start time: .... End time: ....

Find the image that doesn't have a pair and mark it with an X:

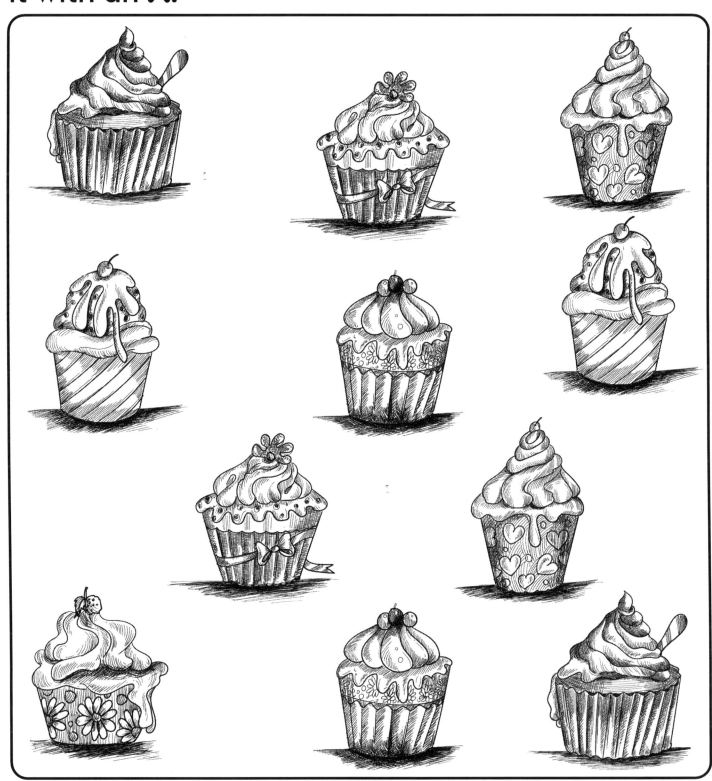

Cognitive Function: **PERCEPTION**

Date: ..../.................../............... Duration: ....

Start time: .... End time: ....

Mark with an **X** the silhouette of the geometric figure that matches the one in the box on the left:

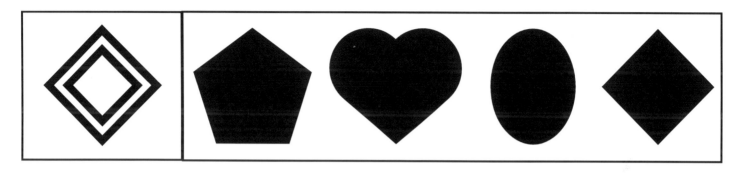

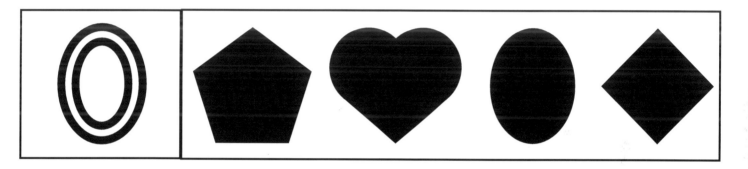

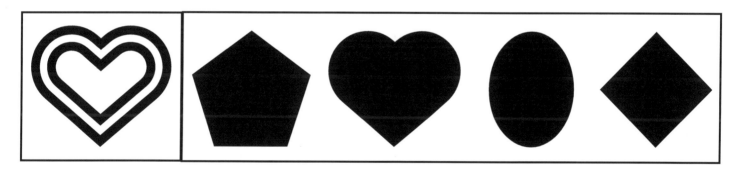

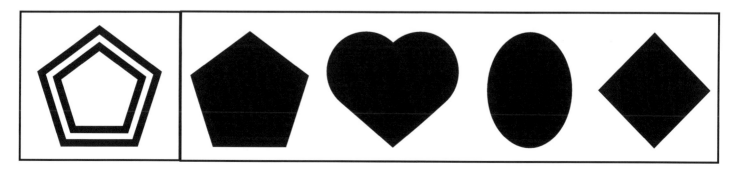

Date: ..../.............../............   Duration: ....

Start time: ....   End time: ....

Copy the picture in the empty grid:

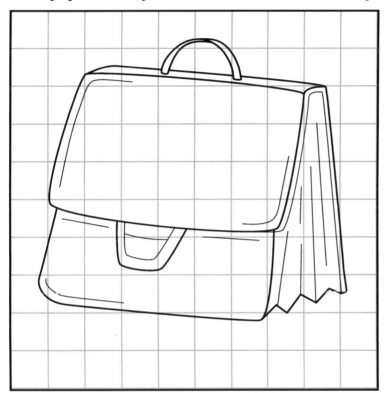

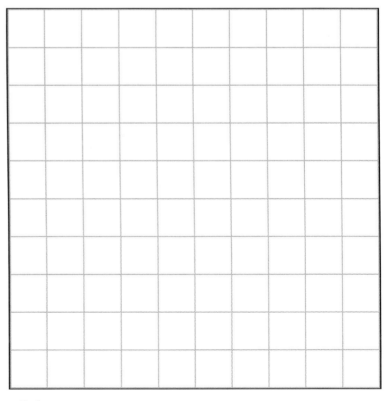

Date: ..../.................../...............   Duration: ....

Start time: ....   End time: ....

Draw a line to connect the opposite word:

hot ◉   ◉ night

fast ◉   ◉ sad

day ◉   ◉ right

happy ◉   ◉ cold

poor ◉   ◉single

left ◉   ◉rich

married ◉   ◉ slow

Cognitive Function: **PERCEPTION**

Date: ..../.............../..............

Duration: ....

Start time: ....

End time: ....

Mark with an **X** the image that is different from the others:

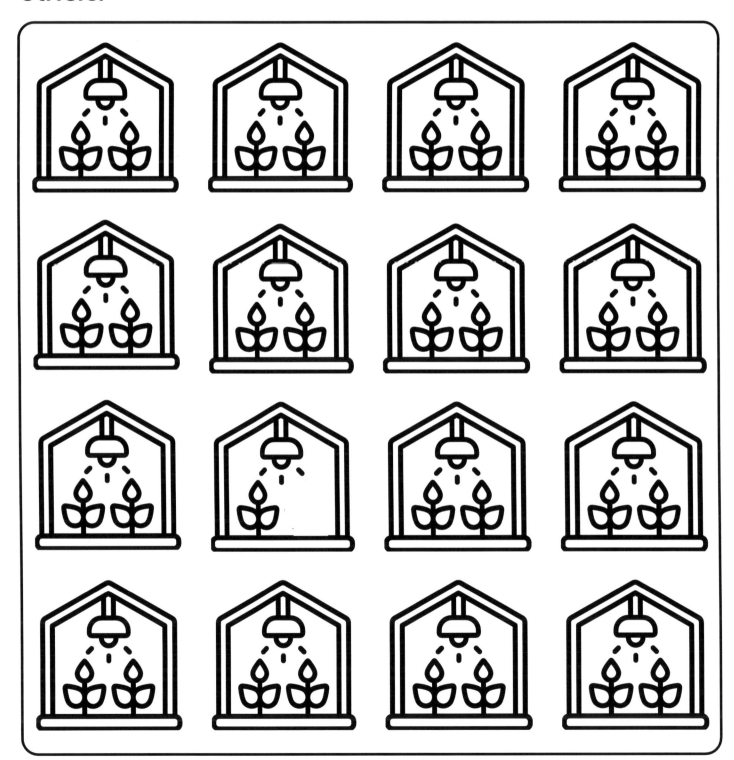

Date: ..../................/...............

Duration: ....

Start time: ....

End time: ....

Connect the equal numbers. The lines cannot cross each other:

3				1
6	2	1		
			3	
6				2

Cognitive Function: **ATTENTION**

Date: ..../.............../.............. Duration: ....

Start time: .... End time: ....

There are 5 (five) differences between the two pictures below. Can you find them?

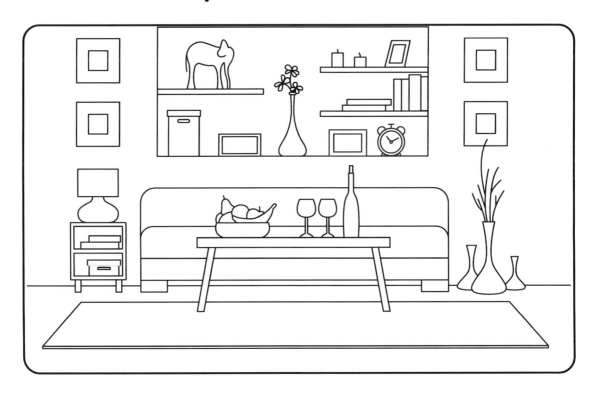

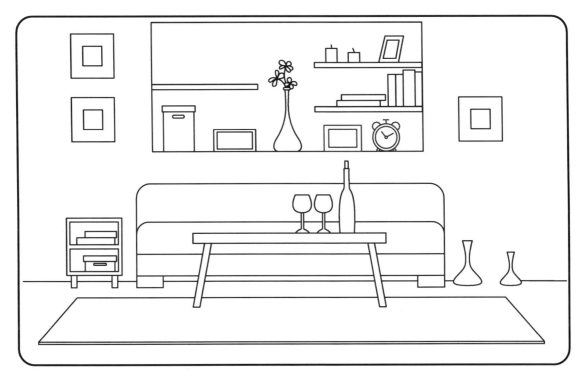

Date: ..../.............../.............   Duration: ....

Start time: ....   End time: ....

Pay close attention and memorize the positions of the letters **X** on the grid. Then go to the next page:

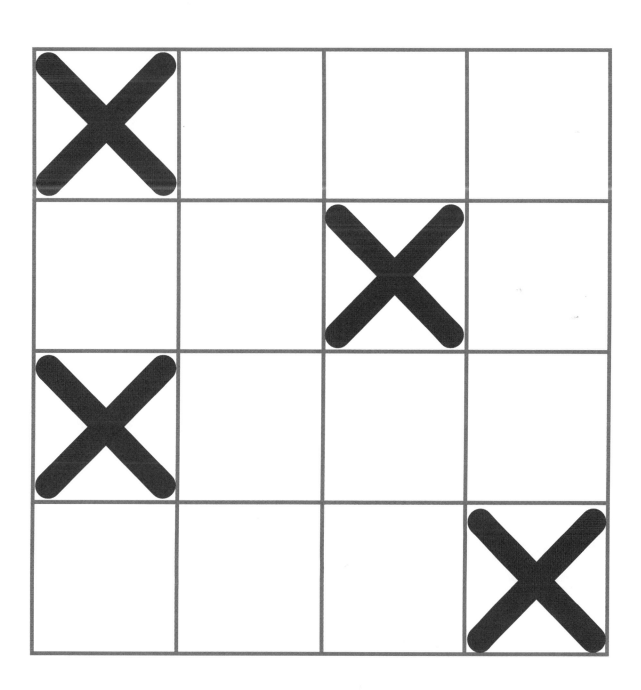

Date: ..../.............../.............   Duration: ....

Start time: ....   End time: ....

On the grid, write the letters **X** where they were placed in the previous page:

Date: ..../ ..../ ....   Duration: ....

Start time: ....   End time: ....

Mark with an **X** the words that have 5 letters or less:

oil	chair	love
noise	bridge	red
eastern	air	brother
four	strong	orange
word	fish	liquid
mouth	soap	day
interest	train	lion
apple	flower	blue
kitchen	river	street

Date: ..../.............../..............   Duration: ....

Start time: ....   End time: ....

Draw a line to connect the image with the box of geometric figures that make it:

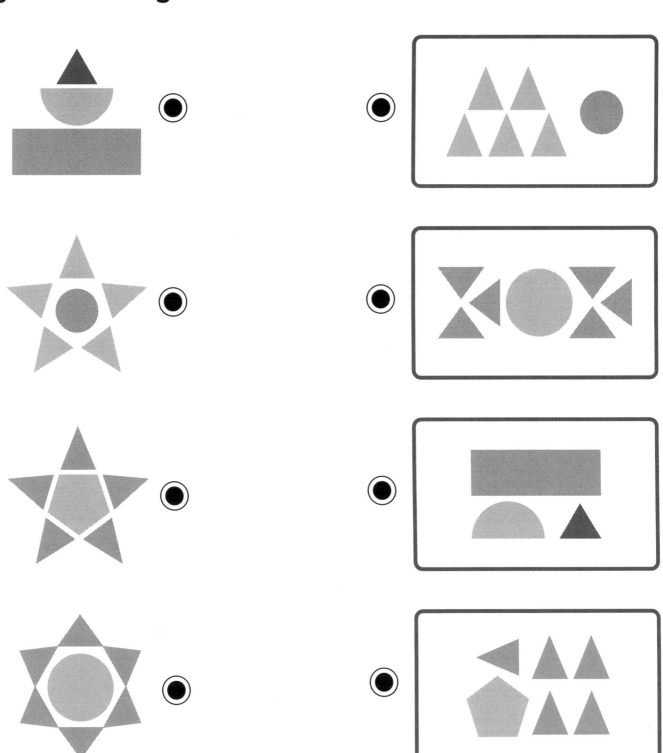

Date: ..../.............../..............   Duration: ....

Start time: ....   End time: ....

Connect the geometric shapes by alternating between circles and rhombuses, following the numerical sequence:

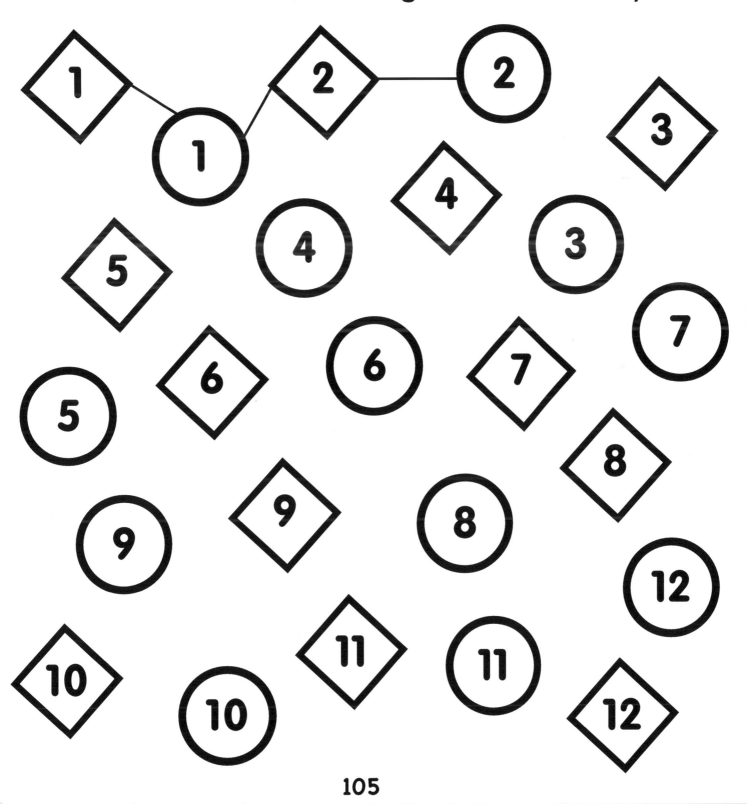

How many figures are there of each geometric figure? Write the number in each box:

Date: ..../.............../.............   Duration: ....

Start time: ....   End time: ....

Complete the maze. Help the pencil reach the sharpener:

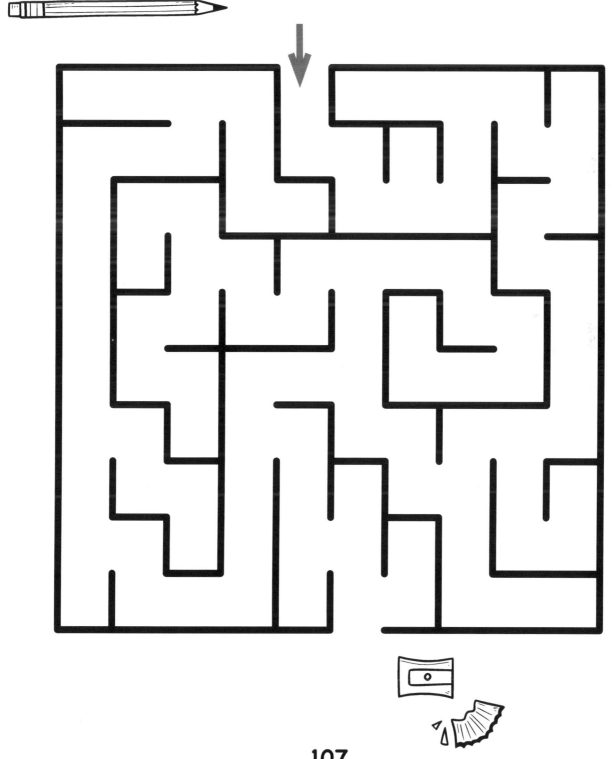

Date: ..../.............../............ Duration: ....

Start time: .... End time: ....

Write the phrase you see on the fence on the lines below:

Experience is the mother of wisdom

....

....

....

....

Date: ..../............../..............   Duration: ....

Start time: ....   End time: ....

Write 3 words that start with the letter in the left circle in each row:

A			
L			
M			
S			
E			
R			

Date: ..../ ..../ ....

Duration: ....

Start time: ....

End time: ....

Arrange and write the number (from 1 to 4) in each circle to create the image in the box:

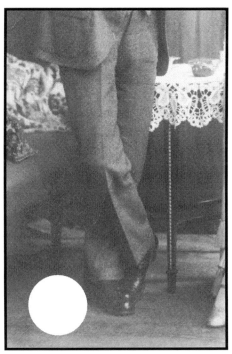
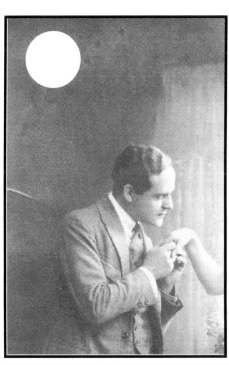
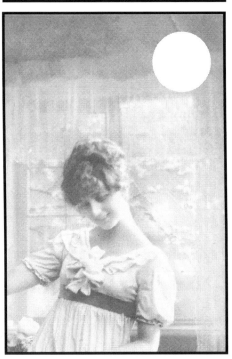
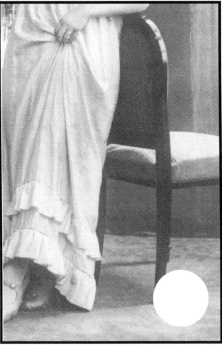
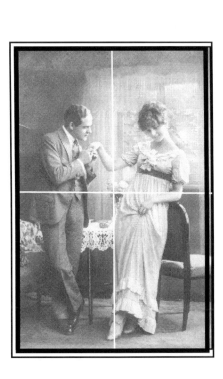

Date: ..../.............../.............

Duration: ....

Start time: ....

End time: ....

Memorize the following letter and number pairs. Then go to the next page:

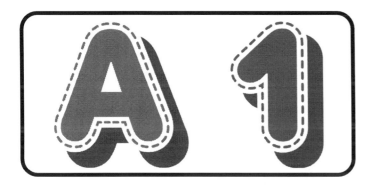

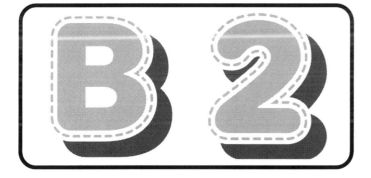

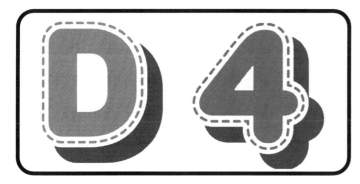

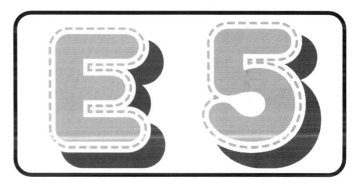

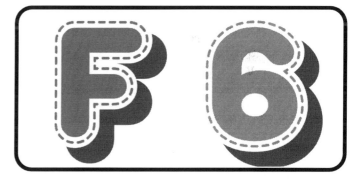

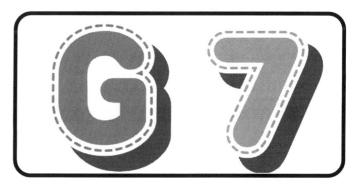

Date: ..../ ..../ ....

Duration: ....

Start time: ....

End time: ....

In each blank box, write the missing number to form the pairs on the previous page:

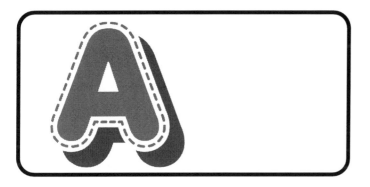

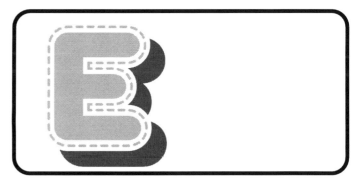

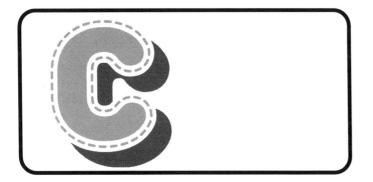

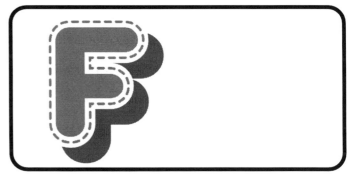

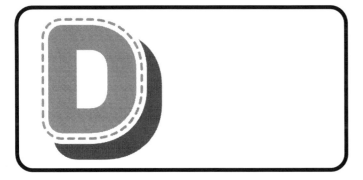

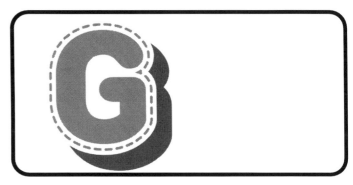

Date: ..../............../.............

Duration: ....

Start time: ....

End time: ....

Look at the following numbers and answer the questions:

28 34 10 15

36 25 13 41

38 19 07 12

What is the largest number? ....

What is the smallest number? ....

Order the numbers from largest to smallest:

....

....

....

ANSWERS

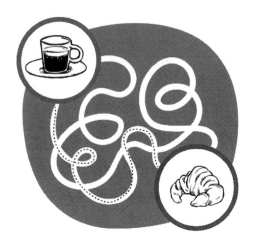

Page 6

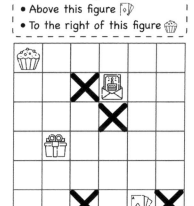

- To the left of this figure ✉
- Below this figure 🍿
- Above this figure 🃏
- To the right of this figure 🧁

Page 7

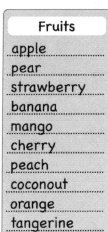

Fruits	Vegetables
apple	onion
pear	garlic
strawberry	lettuce
banana	avocado
mango	carrot
cherry	broccoli
peach	potato
coconout	corn
orange	peas
tangerine	cucumber

Page 8

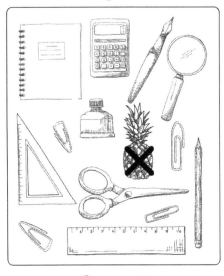

Page 9

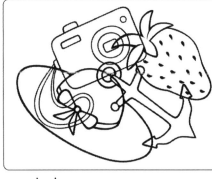

hat
anchor
strawberry
photographic camera

Page 10

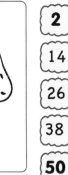

2	4	6	8	**10**	12
14	16	**18**	20	22	24
26	**28**	30	32	34	**36**
38	40	42	**44**	46	48
50	52	54	56	**58**	60
62	64	**66**	68	70	72
74	76	78	80	82	**84**

Page 11

    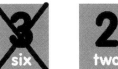 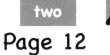

Page 12

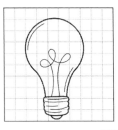

Page 13

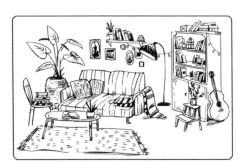

guitar	bush
table	books
coach	cushions
lamp	chair

Page 16

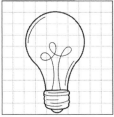

ANSWERS

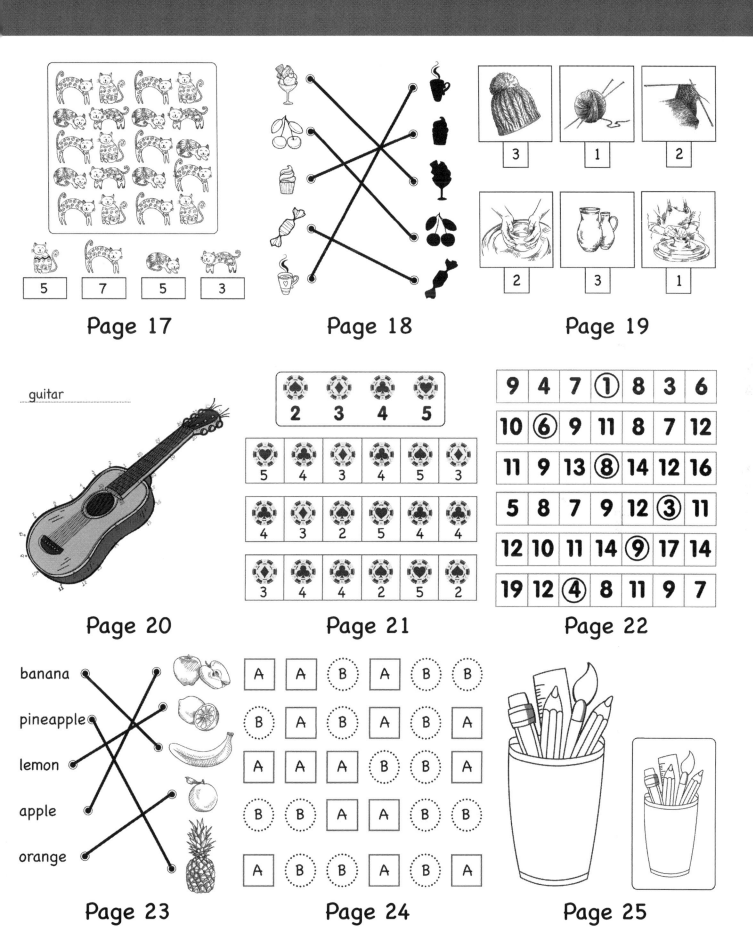

Page 17

Page 18

Page 19

guitar

Page 20

Page 21

Page 22

banana
pineapple
lemon
apple
orange

Page 23

Page 24

Page 25

ANSWERS

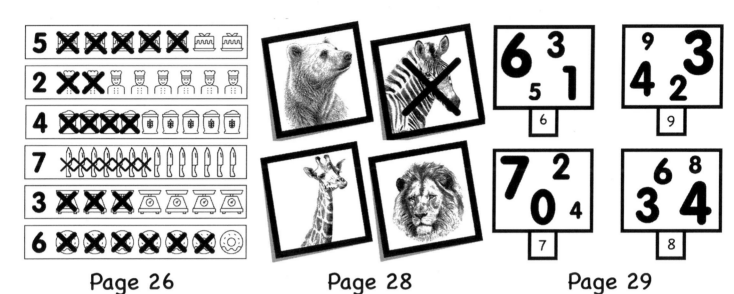

Page 26

Page 28

Page 29

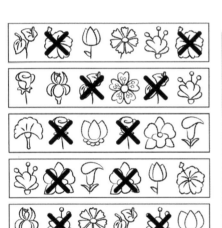

Page 30

Page 31

Page 32

Page 33

Page 34

Page 35

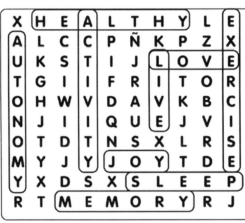

- chair
- candle
- glass of wine
- pear
- table
- books

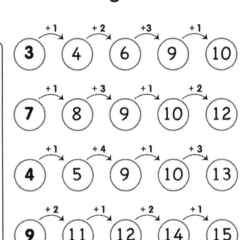

There was once a countryman who possessed the most wonderful goose you can imagine, for every day when he visited the nest, the goose had laid a beautiful, glittering, golden egg.

The countryman took the eggs to the market and soon began to get rich. But it was not long before he grew impatient with the goose because she gave him only a single golden egg a day. He was not getting rich fast enough.

Then one day, after he had finished counting his money, the idea came to him that he could get all the golden eggs at once by killing the goose and cutting it open. But when the deed was done, not a single golden egg did he find, and his precious goose was dead.

Count all the a's and then write the result number in the box. **37**

¿What is the title of the fable?
1. The Ants and the Grasshopper
2. The Goose & the Golden Egg
3. The Wolf and the Shepherd

¿What animal does the countryman have?
The goose

¿What was the material that was made of the goose's eggs?
gold

¿What happened to the goose?
it was killed

ANSWERS

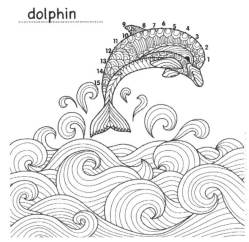

dolphin

Page 36

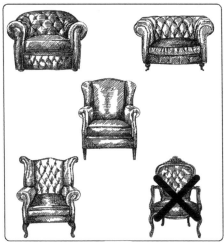

Page 38

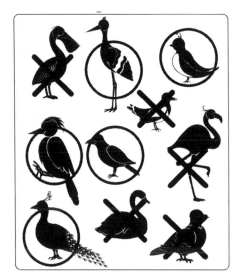

Page 39

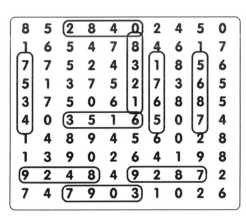

Page 40

iron

radio

mixer

toaster   microwave

blender

Page 41

X	8	X	X	3
2	X	X	1	X
X	X	9	X	5
3	X	X	4	X
X	5	X	X	2
X	1	X	7	X

Page 42

doctor, singer, fireman, scientist, artist, chef, athlete, policeman, mechanic.

chef

policeman

singer

artist

athlete

mechanic

fireman

scientist

doctor

Page 43

	56	22	47	50	71	29	74
	30	68	42	77	25	51	82
	X	X	X	X	59	80	36
23	54	39	65	33	73	X	64	28	76
37	X	X	X	X	X	X	55	31	79
80	X	43	60	27	67	48	24	75	61
44	X	38	53	72	34	40	63	58	26
62	X	X	X	52	45	81			
32	57	70	X	X	78	49			
41	66	35	46	X	X	X			

Page 45

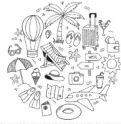

palm	wallet
globe	glasses
hat	chair
suitcase	plane
sun	ice cream

Page 46

117

ANSWERS

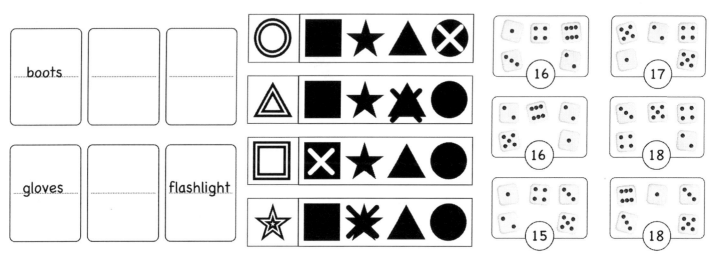

Page 48   Page 49   Page 50

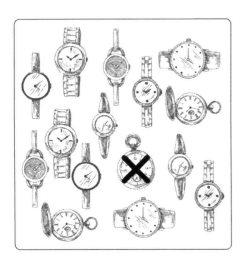

Page 51

No pain — without pain
Don't judge — by its cover
Not gain — no gain
Out of sight — out of mind
Every dog — has its day
Better late — than never
Rome was not built — in one day

Page 52

1 Don't put all your eggs in one basket.

2 Kind words will unlock an iron door.

3 Two wrongs don't make a right.

4 A friend in need is a friend indeed.

5 Curiosity killed the cat.

6 Actions speak louder than words.

Page 53

2	3	1	4	5	6
6	4	5	2	3	1
1	2	4	3	6	5
3	5	6	1	4	2
5	1	3	6	2	4
4	6	2	5	1	3

Page 54

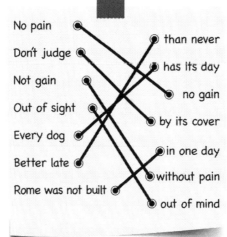

Page 55

The boy is ridding a bike

 The lady is walking a baby in a stroller

The kid is flying a kite

 The boy is playing football

Page 56

ANSWERS

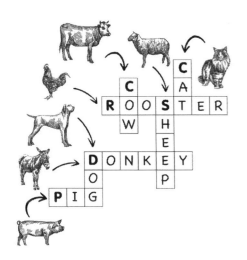

Page 57

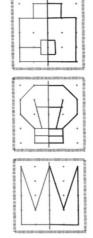 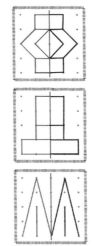

Page 58

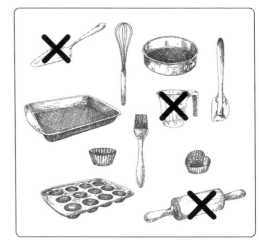

Page 60

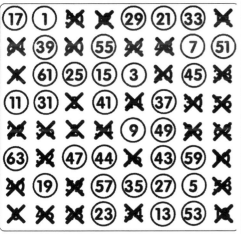

Page 61

1	2	3	4	**5**	6	7	8	9	**10**
11	**12**	13	14	**15**	16	**17**	**18**	21	20
21	22	23	**24**	25	**26**	27	28	**29**	30
31	**32**	33	34	**35**	36	37	38	39	**40**
41	42	**43**	44	45	**46**	47	**48**	49	50
51	**52**	53	54	**55**	56	57	58	**59**	60
61	62	**63**	64	65	**66**	67	**68**	69	**70**
71	72	73	74	**75**	76	77	78	**79**	80
81	**82**	98	**84**	85	86	**87**	88	89	**90**
91	92	**93**	94	95	**96**	97	98	**99**	100

Page 62

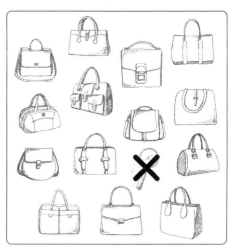

Page 63

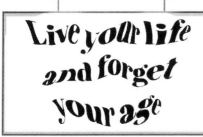

Live your life and forget your
age

Page 64

10	14	18
4	10	17
11	8	20
6	5	16
9	12	15
7	6	11

Page 65

to display the time – to carry money –
for watering plants – to cook food –
to prevent theft – to produce light

for watering   to display   to produce
plants   the time   light

to prevent   to cook food   to carry
theft   money

Page 67

119

ANSWERS

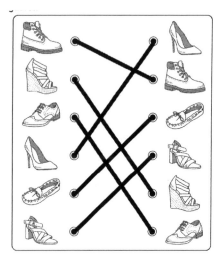

Page 68

- tie
- shoes
- belt
- glasses
- watch
- hat
- keys
- briefcase

Page 70

 3:30
 5:55
 3:50
9:40
2:30
1:45

Page 71

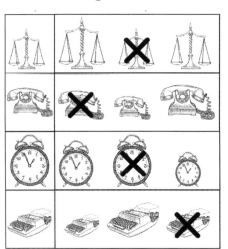

Page 72

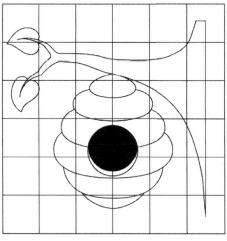

Page 73

F A M I L Y P S L K W
R H F G H J A L K Y I
I O W N B S T Q B V S
E N E R G Y I B V J D
N E N G Q B E K P B O
D Y X Q T R N P M M
S C T Y V N C M P X
H A P P I N E S S T L
I X C O M P A N Y L
P A F F E C T I O N

Page 74

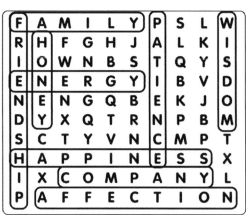

Page 75

6	4	5	3	1	2
3	2	1	6	5	4
5	6	3	2	4	1
2	1	4	5	6	3
4	5	2	1	3	6
1	3	6	4	2	5

Page 76

Page 77

ANSWERS

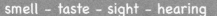

smell - taste - sight - hearing

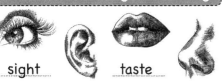

sight .... taste

hearing .... smell

Answer the following questions:

- I can see with my **eyes**
- I can hear with my **ears**
- I can eat with my **mouth**
- I can smell with my **nose**

Page 78

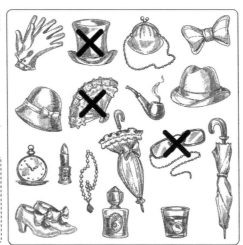

Page 80

```
✗ ✗ 3
7 1 9  = (12)
5 6 2

1 6 9
4 ✗ 8 = (7)
3 7 ✗

4 ✗ 3
5 9 ✗ = (14)
2 7 1

1 2 ✗
4 9 ✗ = (10)
5 6 8
```

```
2 3 1
5 4 ✗ = (15)
6 ✗ 9

2 4 3
1 5 8 = (16)
6 ✗ ✗

6 5 4
2 1 ✗ = (12)
7 8 ✗
```

```
✗ 4 7
2 5 8 = (9)
1 ✗ 9

9 4 ✗
✗ 6 7 = (13)
3 2 1

1 4 7
2 5 ✗ = (11)
✗ 6 9

3 8 5
6 ✗ 9 = (8)
4 ✗ 2
```

Page 81

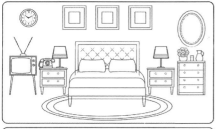

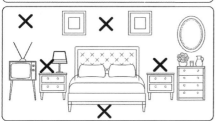

Page 82

dolphin - white - cherry - lion - gray
cat - lemon - blue - dog - apple - bull
- black - coconut - green - grape

COLORS	FRUITS	ANIMALS
white	cherry	dolphin
gray	apple	lion
blue	coconut	dog
black	grape	bull
green	lemon	cat

Page 84

```
1 9 9 0 7 5 9 6 5 0
2 8 0 0 4 (9 4 1 6) 5
3 1 (9 6 4 1 4) 4 0 8
6 7 7 2 0 7 6 5 3 9
1 8 0 6 (2 2 6 8 6) 7
(1) 3 (8 3 4 1 2 8) 5 0
9 0 1 0 2 1 8 2 1 8
4 2 2 3 3 9 1 9 2 5
1 4 7 1 (9 0 3 4) 0 5
5 (1 0 3 7) 6 5 2 0 2
```

Page 85

cat	dog	cow	animals
friday	tuesday	sunday	days
skirt	shirt	pants	clothes
march	may	april	months
green	blue	red	colors
chair	bed	table	furniture
train	boat	plane	transportation
Lisa	Emily	Helen	women's names
daisy	rose	pons	flowers

Page 86

THE FOX & THE GRAPES –Aesop

A Fox One day spied a beautiful bunch of ripe grapes hanging from a vine trained along the branches of a tree. The grapes seemed ready to burst with juice, and the Fox's mouth watered as he gazed longingly at them.

The bunch hung from a high branch, and the Fox had to jump for it. The first time he jumped he missed it by a long way. So he walked off a short distance and took a running leap at it, only to fall short once more. Again and again he tried, but in vain.

Now he sat down and looked at the grapes in disgust.

"What a fool I am," he said. "Here I am wearing myself out to get a bunch of sour grapes that are not worth gaping for."

And off he walked very, very scornfully.

Page 87

CITIES	HOME APPLIANCES
New York	iron
London	fridge
Paris	hairdryer
Miami	dishwasher
San Francisco	Fan

FOOD	CLEANING ITEMS
bread	broom
milk	sponge
cheese	soap
eggs	towel
rice	gloves

Page 88

ANSWERS

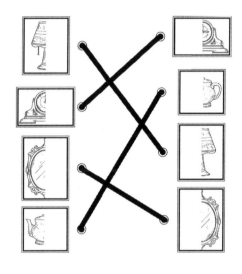

Page 89

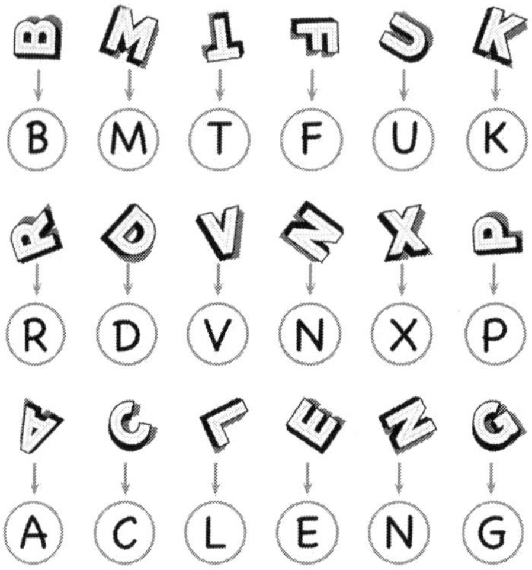

B→B M→M T→T F→F U→K
R→R D→D V→V N→N X→X P→P
A→A C→C L→L E→E N→N G→G

Row 2 circles: B M T F U K
Row 3: R D V N X P
Row 4 circles: R D V N X P
Row 5: A C L E N G
Row 6 circles: A C L E N G

Page 90

yearly	annually
ceiling	roof
tender	soft
expensive	costly
big	large
page	sheet
begin	start
wide	broad
finish	end

Page 91

	A	B	C	D
1	n	e	b	d
2	r	t	g	u
3	f	a	p	k
4	r	n	h	t

great

C2	A4	B1	B3	D4

Page 92

What color is a strawberry?
red

Where do children study?
school

How many months are there in a year?
12

What food comes from cow?
milk and meat

What thing do you use to eat soup?
spoon

What is wine made out of?
grape

Page 93

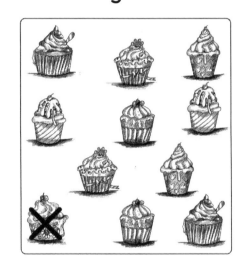

Page 94

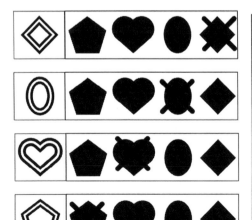

Page 95

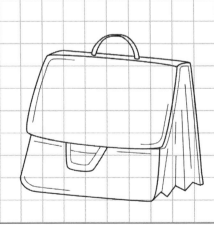

Page 96

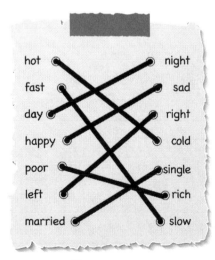

Page 97

hot — cold
fast — slow
day — night
happy — sad
poor — rich
left — right
married — single

122

ANSWERS

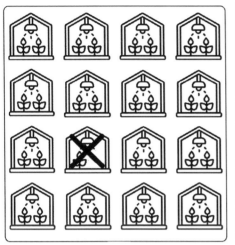

Page 98

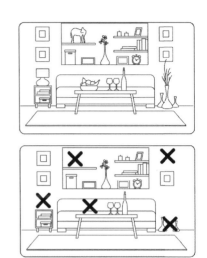

Page 99

Page 100

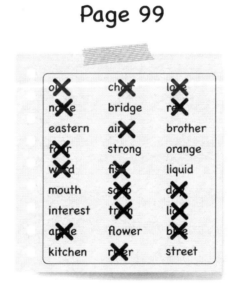

Page 102

Page 103

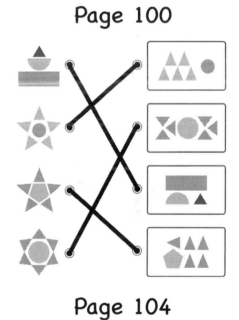

Page 104

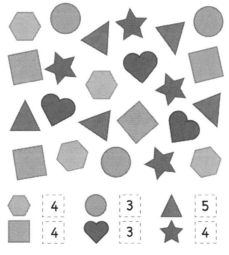

Page 105

Page 106

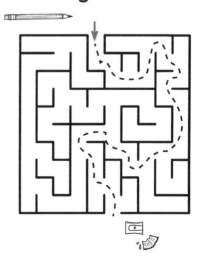

Page 107

ANSWERS

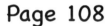

Experience is the mother of
wisdom

Page 108

A	april	Alice	anchor
L	lemon	lake	line
M	menu	middle	milk
S	star	small	short
E	end	eyes	elevator
R	rule	ring	row

Page 109

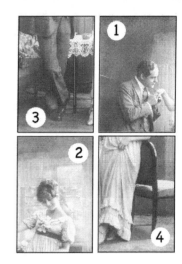

Page 110

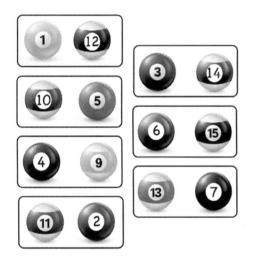

Page 112

(28) (34) (10) (15)

(36) (25) (13) (41)

(38) (19) (07) (12)

What is the largest number? 41
What is the smallest number? 07
Arrange the numbers from greatest to least
41, 38, 36, 34, 28 , 25, 19, 15,
13, 12, 10, 07

Page 113

Thanks
for your support
We hope you enjoyed it
Leaving a review will help us improve
our future products.

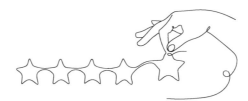

YOUR FEEDBACK MEANS SO MUCH TO US...

We want to sincerely thank you for trusting us by choosing this book. Your support and confidence are the driving force that inspires us to continue developing high-quality products that truly improve people's lives. We hope you enjoy each activity and find moments of joy and connection along the way.

We truly wish you had a great time with this experience! It would mean a lot to us if you could take a moment to leave a review. Not only will it help us as independent authors, but it will also help others find and enjoy these activities too.

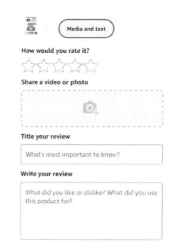

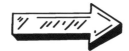

https://amzn.to/479LSeC

Together, we'll make cognitive wellness a reality!

Made in the USA
Columbia, SC
04 June 2025

58635338R00072